W9-CFB-991

LOVE'S FINEST BATTLE

Readers are encouraged to go to www.MissionPointPress.com to contact the author or to find information on how to buy this book in bulk at a discounted rate.

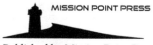

Published by Mission Point Press
2554 Chandler Rd.
Traverse City, MI 49686
(231) 421-9513
www.MissionPointPress.com

Cover photograph by Carrie Nedo of Carrie Lynn's Photography.

ISBN: 978-1-943995-60-8
LoC: : 2018940851

Printed in the United States of America.

Love's Finest Battle

A 30-Year Marriage, Terminal Cancer, and a Husband's Greatest Honor

PAUL WHEELOCK

MISSION POINT PRESS

To the six most incredible and resilient sons a father could hope to have. Becky's beautiful soul lives on in each of them, her legacy forever sealed in their captivating smiles.

CONTENTS

Prologue ... 1

1] When I Stopped Searching ... 7

2] Courting an Angel ... 13

3] The Proposal ... 18

4] The Lion ... 22

5] The Honeymoon Months ... 27

6] Dinner with a Twist ... 32

7] The Greatest Decision Ever ... 35

8] A Line in the Staircase ... 39

9] The Worst Decision Ever ... 43

10] A Parting of the Way ... 51

11] A Sensual Breeze, a Bed Undefiled ... 54

12] Adventures and Misadventures ... 62

13] A Dream Finally Realized ... 65

14] The Bear ... 69

15] Somber Conversations ... 73

16] Goliath ... 77

17] Travel, Sons, and More ... 82

18] A Battle Begins ... 91

Photographs ... 96

19] What a Year! ... 116

20] God's Amazing Grace ... 120

21] The Battle's End in Sight ... 126

22] Let's Plan a Party ... 130

23] A Little Normalcy ... 134

24] One Last Adventure ... 138

25] No Way Out ... 141

26] Wait His Turn ... 149

27] We Made It ... 155

28] Don't Walk, Run! ... 164

29] There Goes My Everything ... 173

30] Notes, A Journal, And the Heart of God ... 176

31] Begging for a Dream ... 182

32] Eternally Yours, My Sweet Love ... 187

Afterword] The Things I've Learned ... 191

About the Author ... 193

Acknowledgements ... 194

LOVE'S FINEST BATTLE

PROLOGUE: THE MONTH AFTER

I woke up as I did any other morning most of the last fifty years of my life. I got out of bed, looked out the window, and headed for the bathroom. On this particular morning, that's where the similarities ended. This time, my eyes were glazed, my heart cold and empty, and what I saw was nothing. No beauty. No definition. No point to anything my brain was processing. Nothing. I made the short walk back to the edge of my bed and sat down, folded my hands on my lap, and felt my head drop, my chin rest on my chest. I was alone. Completely, utterly, hopelessly alone. It had only been five hours since saying goodbye to my sweet bride, my best friend, and the only love of my life. My Becky.

The last twenty-seven years of loving God and sensing Him in my life seemed a distant memory at this point. I was struggling to even breathe, let alone comprehend what had just happened and why. I was quite certain He wasn't anywhere to be found.

As I sat there in the deepest, darkest despair I'd ever encountered, unable to speak or think clearly, and feeling that my heart could stop at any second, the one who said He would never leave me or forsake me broke the silence. He began to deal with that very thing ... my heart. You see, it's there, in the *heart* of man,

that God lives and functions. Not in our brains, where we ana-
lyze and question, reason and doubt, but in our hearts. That's
where faith lives. That's where the issues of life flow.

He began to show me a metaphor for the hours, days, months,
and years leading up to this morning. Surprisingly, He showed
me a football. Yep, that oval-shaped, stitched-leather icon of the
gridiron. He compared the small football to the limited number
of people Becky would have influenced and affected in a powerful way had she been perfectly healthy and lived long ... even to
a hundred.

Odd metaphor, right?

But then He showed me the bigger picture. He revealed that
because Becky had endured cancer these past nine years, and
because we had used a blog to diligently document and share
with stark transparency her brave fight, her true impact by the
end of her life, at age 48, was that of a football *stadium. Thousands of people now knew her story, knew of her bravery, knew of
her triumph.*

I chewed on this wisdom for over thirty minutes, still at the
edge of the bed. But I remained distracted. Still numb. Reflexes
kicked in. I began going about my routine. Feeding the dogs, letting them out, taking my small number of morning pills—blood
pressure medicine and a few supplements—and starting a pot of
coffee. But I wandered around the house for what seemed like
hours, doing nothing, really. I found myself walking in circles.
At one point, I carried a napkin around in my hand for a good
twenty minutes as I tried to find my way to the garbage can only
a few feet away.

There's a reason so many grief experts advise you to *not* make
any major decisions immediately after a loved one's death.
Instead, you should do as much as possible to prepare before,
and then make sure someone is around to help after. The overwhelming sense of nothingness was paralyzing. I had to force
myself to breathe, to walk, and to think. All I wanted to do was
lie down, exhale, and be with her.

Partway through the day, I realized I needed to go to the funeral home with some essentials for the service. Thankfully, I had already gone through thousands of pictures we had taken over that thirty-year span, picking out a couple of hundred so the director could make a slide show. I had already selected the outfit I thought she would look best in for the visitation, and I had written her obituary. There is a certain peace and benefit in preparing for the loss of someone, especially the woman who I had been "one" with for thirty years.

Our son Stephen was home for the week, and so I hollered at him from downstairs and asked if he'd join me in the ride to our little town in Leelanau County, Michigan, called Suttons Bay. "Sure, dad," he said. And off we went.

As I drove down the road, I realized I wasn't concentrating on anything other than Becky, including the road. Not good. I looked at Stephen. "You know, you probably shouldn't be riding with me today," I said. He chuckled a nervous laugh but knew quickly that I wasn't joking. I asked him to help me pay attention and speak up if it looked like I had checked out mentally. The twenty-five-minute ride went by in seconds, it seemed. I did my thing at the funeral home and headed home. It was the first time I'd been gone from the house in the hours following her death. Pulling back in the drive was gut wrenching. She wasn't there, and she wouldn't be there the next time, or the time after that, or ever. And that was more than I could bear. Once I was alone again, I lost it. I collapsed on the bed, wailing in pain, soaking my pillow in tears. For the first time in my entire life, I was totally and utterly alone. Now what? But more important: Why?

For the last thirty-two years, Becky had been the "why" in every decision, every plan, every dream, and every hope. And without her, the "why" was painfully and noticeably gone. Purpose seemed a thing of the past, and no matter how hard I tried that first couple of weeks, I couldn't even begin to imagine my life beyond the next thirty seconds, forget the next thirty years. I was going through the motions. I knew the "what" to do. That list was quite long. In fact, it had doubled in size now that Becky was no longer here. The problem remained the "why." And without the "why," what difference would any of it make anyway?

In fact, over time, my focus would eventually shift from struggling to understand *why* this all happened to *how* I would respond because of it. That's the test each of us faces at some point when dealing with the deepest grief. How will we handle things? How will we cope? How will we love? In short, how will we take these cards we were dealt and use them to either bring glory to God and reflect His love, grace and mercy, or blame God and others and allow the circumstances to engulf us ... to take us down a road with a much more destructive end.

．　．　．　．

It's been just over a month, and I'm writing this prologue from the RV that I bought for our trip out West just nine months ago. Becky and I were able to go to the Grand Canyon and Arches National Park and take about a seventeen-day vacation together, just the two of us and our pair of Miniature Pinschers. This is the first trip I've taken from home since her passing. The ride to Indiana was the worst, most depressing, and soul-crushing road trip I've ever been on in my life. I love to drive. I love road trips. At least I used to. It was all I could do to glance over to the passenger-side mirror. Every time I did, I noticed again that she wasn't there. It's hard to drive with tears spilling from your eyes.

Our oldest son Tim is running the family business, immersing himself in work as his way of dealing with the grief. Because he's doing a fantastic job, I've been able to come and visit some great friends whom you'll get to know later. Ultimately, I'll make my way over to Illinois to be a part of the birth of our second oldest son's child. Andy and Jessica passed their due date just last week. Soon, I'll have a new grandchild. I was never supposed to be a single grandpa. Becky's two greatest joys in life were our marriage and our kids, and she was ready to be the greatest grandma ever. I will never get over the lost opportunity to witness that.

Today at church in Indiana, I met a new friend after striking up a conversation about my loss and my journey. He said he was hoping to be the first to die in his marriage, so his wife could continue on and live her life. I told him I had felt the same way myself, many months ago. "Lord, take me," I prayed. "Let me take her place." But I no longer feel that way. I explained to him my changed thinking: Even though I'm in the midst of unimaginable sorrow and grief, I said, every time I share our story, especially the details of the final couple of weeks, I catch myself finding more and more reasons to be incredibly grateful to God. The fact is, I said, Becky graduated to Heaven first; she is not left here to deal with this kind of agonizing and paralyzing sorrow. Her love for me was as deep, if not deeper, than my love for her, and had I died first, the pain and suffering for her would have been devastating. I'm glad she got to Heaven first. Maybe that's just being selfish on my part. I don't know. I don't think so.

I've talked to countless people with similar stories of loss—so many widows and widowers. What strikes me is that they all, without fail and no matter the length of time since their loss, tear up and become noticeably emotional about their experience. I'm now realizing that grief will be my lifelong companion. Sure, it'll change in severity and timing, length and depth, but nevertheless, it's here to stay. The sooner I settle that in my heart, the sooner I can move on.

I'm also learning that the secret to picking up the pieces and finding any semblance of life's joys is to first give myself permission to live again. I have to acknowledge the loss ... the dreams unfulfilled ... the fairy-tale love story unfinished. But I must also acknowledge that unless I give myself the freedom to move on, I'm destined to stay stuck in this pit of self-destructive quicksand forever, never to love anything or anyone again. Becky, in her wisdom, asked me to make this promise of freedom to her, and I never did. But now I understand why she thought it was so important.

In this book, I'm certainly not going to try to lecture on the right or wrong way to grieve. I'm simply going to share our story, as I've done for nine years now through our blog, as transparently as I can in the hopes that at least a few can find some comfort, some joy, some laughs, some gut checks, and some hope in the journey that was laid out before us and now just me.

Perhaps what God said was a stadium can grow to two stadiums, or three, or even more. But if not, that's okay, too.

So, in these pages I live the journey again, from beginning to end. I share all of the incredible details that made Becky the greatest prize a man could be given. I share the kind of love story that our sons now dream of for themselves. Our love story was just that ... love. No pride, envy, jealousy, or ego. Just tons and tons of love, mixed with sorrow, pain, suffering, and crushed dreams.

Our story was, simply, amazing.

Thank you for letting us share it.

1] WHEN I STOPPED SEARCHING

It was the early 1980s, and I was one of tens of thousands of teenage boys across the country looking for "perfect love." You name the pretty girl, and I probably had a crush on her. I was a homebody by nature, spending most of my childhood hanging out with my parents and their friends or at my grandparents' house. I was never a very adventurous guy, not much into sports, and most definitely not into the party scene that seemed to be everywhere. At the time, it appeared that only the guys in sports or those who partied had the pretty girlfriends and all the fun.

I had a job, a car, good grades, a gentleman's approach, and lots of time, but no girl. In fact, I had never really been on a serious date. There was that one trip to the movies with a girl in my bowling league. And an almost-date with a girl who wanted to tear my clothes off after a fast drive through the woods in her parents' car. But that was it. (I quickly ended the fast-driver date and told my dad the whole story the next day). Then there was the homecoming dance when I—now a senior—made the mistake of taking a *freshman*. What was I thinking? I couldn't get her home fast enough. We didn't dance a single song. I felt like

I was hanging out with my little sister—though I think I would have had at least some fun with my sister. It was a horrible night.

The problem was—*my* problem was—I didn't think any girl who I found interesting would be interested in me. I was boring, not very athletic, and way too old fashioned for the '80s ladies.

I spent most of my time with my new best friend Mark, who I met when I was a sophomore and he a senior. He and I were like kindred spirits and became inseparable my last two years of school. Mark and I had a ton in common, not the least of which was an overwhelming desire to send all girls packing so we could forget about them. We were tired of the drama and the pressure to be perfect male specimens in order to get even a glance. So, we did our own thing. Mark played the guitar and I the drums. We spent hours jamming to Journey, 38 Special, and his favorite band at the time, Cheap Trick. Those were two very fun years; they went by quickly but, oh, so perfectly.

Sometime in my junior year, my parents started attending a nearby church. They would take my sisters and I along, and our entire family eventually fell in love with the pastor and his wife and enjoyed attending there. It was during that year that I half-heartedly gave my heart to Jesus and asked him to make something of my life. I sure had no idea which way to go with it. College? Girls? Job? At 17, I had no answers, but I knew I would need to make some decisions soon. It was shortly after then that I made one of the most God-centered decisions of my life: I would not pursue any girl. Instead, I would wait for God to bring a girl to me. I believed that God knew my heart, and that He had created someone, somewhere, who was thinking, wondering, and maybe even praying for the same thing I was.

I read in scripture where God created Eve as a helpmate to Adam, someone to complete what was lacking in him and to be a partner ... a spiritual companion; to become one flesh in every sense of the word. So, yeah, basically I was waiting on a miracle. But I didn't care. I'd spent too much time dreaming about the perfect match. I had failed in my attempts to dance with pretty girls at the teen dances. I had thrown long and starry-eyed glances across rooms, to no effect. Nothing got me a date. Instead, I was a lonely, esteem-deprived, hopeless, teenage boy who really thought he wasn't good enough. So, what did I have to lose by asking God to take away this burden? Not a thing.

I was working at Sugar Loaf, a resort in Leelanau County, at the time. The county is in the northwest corner of Michigan's Lower Peninsula. When I was off work, I was usually with Mark in nearby Traverse City, hiking, or attending a dance just so we could hang out with the disc jockey, Larry Pleva, or at Mark's house (or mine) visiting with our parents. We also loved to shoot guns, hunt, and—our favorite activity—cruise Front Street in Traverse with our car stereos blasting and our ears ringing. We were busy all of the time; it was great.

One evening in late fall of 1984, Mark was working and I was bored. I wanted to go to the teen dance in Cedar but didn't want to go alone. I loved helping Larry, the disc jockey; he let me and a few other guys pick the music, run the lights, and often times we'd help set up and tear down. Kind of like his roadies. Anyway, I wanted to go this night, so I called my cousin Sherry in Traverse City.

She was my age, and she and I had grown very close over the past several years. We were great friends and loved hanging out when we got the chance. I was happy to hear her say yes. I headed into town, picked her up, and we drove to the small village of Cedar. The dances usually lasted about four hours and were really quite fun. Sherry and I danced to almost every song together. And yes, even some of the slow songs. No, we weren't kissing cousins … just really great friends. After the dance, I took Sherry home and headed to my house and to bed so I'd be ready for work early the next morning. Little did I know, though, that there was a certain Suttons Bay girl at the dance who was drawn to me but couldn't bring herself to say hi because she thought I was with my girlfriend.

(*Quick side note*: If you're taking your beautiful cousin to a dance, and you've asked God to bring the perfect girl to you in the meantime, you may be sabotaging the whole process. Just saying.)

It would be a few months before this certain girl would figure out that Sherry was my cousin. But then, just as I had prayed, God stepped in, bringing this precious gift my way. Here's what happened: Her best friend was dating one of my friends and classmates at the time. The Suttons Bay girl decided to write me a letter. She gave it to her friend, who passed it to her boyfriend— my classmate—who delivered it to me in computer class. It was early January, my senior year, 1985.

What a day! The letter was two full pages, front and back. I can still remember how I felt reading it. This girl thought I was superman. Not literally, of course, but in every other sense. She thought I was gorgeous. She thought I was a great dancer. She was very excited to find out from her friend that I was with my cousin that night and not on a date. With my classmate's help, she had also added that she wanted to "jump my bones"—a phrase I would remind her of for decades to come, and often get a blush in return.

She included her phone number in the letter and asked me to give her a call. Boy, was I nervous. At this point, I didn't think "this must be God's answer to my prayer." Instead, I was apprehensive about it all, to be honest. I mean, really, after all the shut downs and cold shoulders, how could a girl be this interested in me? No way, I thought. But there was no way I *wasn't* going to dial that number.

I'll never forget that phone call. Mostly we talked about our connections with our friends, and how the letter exchange came about. We talked about dances and the fact that she had noticed me back in Cedar. But it wasn't the words themselves that caught my attention. What got my heart racing and the butterflies in my belly twirling was her voice. She had a certain *way* with her words, like a Southern drawl but not that pronounced. In an instant, I fell in love with her voice.

We talked on the phone almost every day for a week or two, and planned a time and place to meet. We decided on the teen dance scheduled for January 18, 1985, at St. Rita's Hall in Maple City, which is just up the road from Cedar. The disc jockey was, of course, our friend and music hero, who actually went by the name of "Larry Pleva and the Sound Machine." I was going to get there late, because I had to play in the pep band for our home basketball game at Glen Lake.

That night, my heart and mind were nowhere near that gymnasium. All I could think about was the girl. Keep in mind that I had no idea what she looked like, how tall she was, color of hair, nothing. I just knew her voice. My friend, Jack, had met her once in Suttons Bay when he was picking up his girlfriend, Teri; he said I'd like her. But that was it. No photos. Just our phone calls. I was nervous, anxious, excited, and scared to death.

Finally, halftime of the game came around, and we were free to go. I couldn't get out of the gym fast enough. It was usually only about a five-minute drive to Maple City but a little longer this night because of heavy snow. I walked in the door, paid my cover, and spotted Jack across the room. He was sitting with two girls. Teri was one; I assumed the other was my mystery date.

Very carefully, very nervously, I walked across the room, said "Hey" to Jack, and exchanged a few words about the weather, trying to be cool and slow my beating heart. Then came the introduction. Jack motioned me toward the girl, and we shook hands. We chatted for just a bit, and a slow song started to play. I thought, *Of all things, our first dance would have to be to a slow song!*

The room was dark, but the dance floor was illuminated by beams of colorful lights timed to the music. That was the main reason we headed out there, so we could actually see each other. As my dad had taught me, I very gently—like a gentleman—

placed my hands on her sides. She put hers on my shoulders, and we began swaying to the music. And amazingly, fantastically, in just five minutes, the date was over. Over? Yes ... because by the end of that first song, we had fallen madly, deeply, completely, most assuredly in love. Impossible? Only in fairy tales? Only in the movies? All I can say is that after those five minutes, there was one thing we both knew: God had brought us together, and we would be together for the rest of our lives. By the time the next song started, we were no longer on a date. We were on a relationship-building adventure.

After that night, I would see her every day for weeks and weeks, with only a few exceptions. And on those days that I didn't, we talked forever on the phone. We couldn't go a day, sometimes an hour, without hearing each other's voice. Soon, we talked about a wedding ... we absolutely knew it would happen. In such a short amount of time, this girl had come crashing into my life, and my heart was on fire with every word she spoke, with every glance she gave.

I couldn't stop thinking about her. All I wanted to do at my job was jump in my car and drive as fast as I could to be with her. She lived a good twenty-minute ride from my house and thirty minutes from work, depending on snowfall. Didn't matter though. I would have driven hours and days to be with her. She had captured my heart, my soul, my mind. My life had almost instantly become incredibly focused, full of purpose, in ways I never imagined possible.

I didn't know the details yet, I hadn't met her family yet—I knew little about her outside of dancing and phone calls—but I knew one thing for certain: I was going to marry this girl as soon as humanly possible.

She—Becky Boone—would be my best friend, my wife, my one and only love for all of eternity. Of this I had no doubt.

2] COURTING AN ANGEL

can remember the ride to Becky's home from St. Rita's Hall like it was ten minutes ago. Jack and Teri were in the front seat and Becky and I in the backseat of his Chrysler K-car station wagon.

What I'm about to tell you goes against everything I ever taught my kids, and it probably wasn't the most appropriate thing to have done as a Christian. But knowing what I know now, guess what? I wouldn't have changed a thing. That is, man oh man, did I love kissing her—from the very first moment our lips locked. Call it hormones, first love, fate, whatever you want. All I know is that in a span of a few hours, I had completely fallen for this girl; she consumed every molecule of my being, from the top of my head to the soles of my feet. When you know, you just know.

We stood at her doorway for what seemed like hours. Jack was very patient as he waited in the car to take me back to my car in Maple City. It was cold, snowy, but I was on fire, and nothing could put the flame out.

One evening, a week later, I met her parents. As we visited, her dad, Bud, got a phone call from Becky's grandma, his mom. Bea and Jake Boone lived next door, and she was calling to let Bud know she had heard a loud crash near the barns. Bud threw his coat on, as did we, and we ran out the door. We found a caved-in roof from the heavy snow; livestock were trapped in the rubble. This had turned into an interesting first meeting! We worked until well after midnight removing debris and freeing animals, and I ended up spending the night and had breakfast with them the next morning.

Breakfast was an interesting experience as well. I won't share details. Let's just say the issue was her mom's cooking. So much an issue, in fact, that it had me briefly—stupidly—rethinking my decision to live the rest of my life with Becky.

Now, I love Becky's mom—because, well, she's Becky's mom. But after growing up in a home with a mother who could make the most basic ingredients taste like a four-star dinner, and having a grandmother who was equally amazing in the kitchen, I was a bit concerned. After all, daughters usually learn that sort of thing from their moms. I wasn't sure I could spend the rest of my life eating like this, and I knew we'd both be in trouble if the cooking fell to me. (Oh, I could cook. I just didn't like it much and knew if it were up to me, the menu would be bland and redundant.)

It didn't take long to learn that Becky was a fine cook. She knew her way around the kitchen, having spent lots of time with her grandma and an aunt or two. Becky told me early on that she paid close attention to folks in her life who could cook, because she knew she'd be on her own someday—likely with someone special—and she wanted to eat good-tasting food. Keep in mind that thirty years ago, eating out wasn't anywhere near as popular or doable as it is now. And guys just didn't cook as much as they do now.

Over the next weeks and months, I would spend a ton of time at Becky's house, helping her with chores, playing with her baby goats, getting annoyed at the older goats, and sneaking off to the barn every chance I could to kiss my girlfriend.

I now wonder how many couples can remember the first time their lover spoke the words, "I love you." I can, like it was yesterday. We were sitting on the couch on the east wall of her parent's living room, just hanging out with her family, watching and playing with her dogs. We sat as close to each other as possible without causing her dad too much concern. I had my right arm around her, and my left hand was holding her left hand on our laps. She reached over with her right hand and tapped my right knee. One tap, then four taps, finishing with three taps.

Tap ... tap tap tap tap ... tap tap tap.

I remember looking at her with a funny, question-mark kind of grin. She did it again, and then again. After about the fourth or fifth time, the light clicked on in my knucklehead brain, and my heart exploded in my chest. *I ... love ... you.* This was the first woman outside my family to share these words with me, but this was completely different. A different kind of love. And no, she didn't speak the words, but I heard her loud and clear. She told me later that she had to let me know, right then and there, and that was the only way to do it and not cause a stir.

From that moment on, we almost drilled a hole into each other's knees from tapping. When Becky spoke those words for years to come, she would always start with a question. She would get my attention, look me straight in the eye, and say "guess what?" Without hesitation, knowing what was coming, I would answer, "what?" And each time, after the taps, she would smile and say, "I love you." And to this day, every time I think about that, my throat seizes and tears flow. Words can't describe how precious that was to me, and how I regret the few times I thought it was silly.

So, for the first time in high school, I had a date for both homecoming and prom. I had to be the happiest and luckiest guy in the world. I wasn't attending these with my girlfriend. I was attending these with my future wife. We weren't married yet ... wouldn't be for a while. But in my heart she was my wife, and I was her husband, and we had our eyes set on that reality.

Now, obviously, in terms of a physical relationship, we weren't married. But boy oh boy, sometimes we wished we were—right then and there. I remember while dancing with her, I couldn't take my eyes off her smile ... unless she was wearing a low-cut shirt or gorgeous prom dress. Then my eyes struggled with gravity. Not my fault, really. God is the one who created her that way.

In fact, it was nearly impossible to keep our hands off each other. But we did, sort of. Oh yeah, we pushed the boundaries to the farthest reaches ... no doubt. But we never allowed ourselves to take that final step. We talked about it all the time, and we remember agreeing on many occasions that there was no way we were going to ruin the most glorious wedding night a couple could imagine. I wanted to carry her over the threshold with butterflies in my stomach the size of eagles ... to experience the anticipation that only that kind of moment can bring. She agreed.

That, by the way, would be a conversation I would have repeatedly with our sons years later as they began dealing with hormones. You only get to give your virginity to one person, ever, I said. Once it's gone, it's gone. You can never take it back; you can't rewrap it and give it to another as a new gift.

Like the taps on the knee, Becky did something else that would always make me feel the most special. Anytime I drove up to meet her somewhere and got out of the car, she would make eye contact, then come running. She wouldn't stop until she was completely off the ground in my arms, squeezing me with everything she had. That was always followed by the most amazing kisses. I was smitten for sure; life was as good as I dreamed it could ever be.

One night, on my way to one of Becky's 4-H meetings, the radio blurted some news that would take the wind out of us for a few days. 4-H was a huge part of Becky's life. She had been involved for years. The meeting, on April 14, 1986, was focused on planning a trip to North Carolina that summer. She invited me to come along on the trip, so she asked me to come to the meeting. The radio said we had just bombed Libya, and that people had died. Back then, this was a big deal. I was 18 and eligible for the draft. If this escalated, well, what then? We might be separated and never see each other again. It took our breath away that night and weighed on us for several days, until it was clear we weren't going to war.

The other big thing happening then was that Mark and I were seeing each other less and less. Part of me struggled with that. He and I had been joined at the hip for a long time; Becky was now in that spot. He didn't have a girlfriend, and hanging out with us was awkward for him. He worked a lot, and he and I would still hang out when Becky was working. But most of my free time was spent with just her. He understood, and he and I remained very good friends.

I can't emphasize enough how important it was that Becky was now my best friend. My need for other friends or hobbies had disappeared overnight in January, and Becky was now my only focus. For 32 years, that would be the secret weapon in our amazing marriage. We were, and always would be, each other's everything.

3] THE PROPOSAL

t's May, 1986, and we're at a jeweler's showroom in Acme feeling goosebumps as we hold hands and pick out wedding rings. We knew sixteen months earlier we'd be doing this, and since Becky was a senior and would be graduating—and I had already graduated the year prior—we could finally make it official. The whole world was going to know that Becky was to be Mrs. Wheelock and make me *the most blessed man ever*. I know, a lot of guys say those kinds of things. But this was the real deal. There are seven billion people on the planet, and about three billion of those are men. And yet God decided that I would have the privilege and honor of taking Becky by the hand and spend the rest of my life with her, loving her and honoring my vows. To this day, that blows my mind—that He trusted me enough to be that guy.

We had the rings, but we had decided an official engagement would come later. Becky still had to graduate, for starters. Graduation day came, and I had my 1980 Buick Regal all shined and ready for the ride. I picked Becky up—she was dressed in her graduation garb—and headed for Suttons Bay for the ceremony. I had deliberately arrived at her house early, and we left for the school early as well. Unknown to her or anyone else, I had planned to stop along the way. I could hardly contain myself.

For reasons I won't detail too deeply, I didn't plan to ask Becky's dad for permission to marry her. Both of our sets of parents would go on to divorce over the next several years—Becky's right away and mine later. We both sensed there would be problems ahead in her parents' relationship. Maybe that's why it felt okay to skip the "dad's-permission" thing. We just didn't see them as the ideal models for our marriage.

On the other hand, Becky and I loved to visit my great grandparents, Millard and Vera Hartman, during those courting days. Here they were, married, 50-plus years. They would sit and hold hands, and he would take care of her every need. She was confined to a chair most of the day and couldn't do much for herself in those last few years, but my grandpa took care of her, almost always sporting a smile.

I remember telling Becky often that I was going to be just like him and take care of her until we both grew old. We planned on beating their record; we'd be married at least sixty years. In hindsight, thank goodness we had these great examples of marriage and faithfulness—and that we could see how wedding vows, in all their wonder, can be tested later in life when the brutality of aging or illness kicks in and threatens to destroy hopes and dreams.

As for our parents ... well, they would go on to damage their love stories. They would allow things to enter in and take away what Becky and I would spend every day cherishing. We would see the signs of trouble as time went on but could only sit and watch as their vows were broken and their lives forever changed.

By the way, for the record, I feel divorce is *not* the unpardonable sin that so many people say it is. God will forgive; He moves on with us and for us.

Anyway, back to graduation day. I pulled the car into one of our favorite parking spots, the boat launch across M-22 from Hilltop Road, along Grand Traverse Bay. We had spent countless evenings there, talking, walking the beach, sitting on the dock, holding hands, kissing, and making out like there was no tomorrow. I parked the car and shut it down. I knew she wondered what we were doing; she thought we were just stopping to smooch some more, or maybe talk about the details of her graduation.

I didn't get down on one knee as many do. The weather was rainy and the ground damp. The car had a sunroof, though, that lit up the inside with natural light. I turned to face her, asked her to close her eyes, and I took her left hand. I could sense her heart rate increasing; she thought this would happen much later, in the summer or fall. I grasped the engagement ring in my right hand as I held her left hand, then asked her to open her eyes. As she did, I slipped the ring on her finger and instantly asked her, my voice trembling, to marry me.

It was the most amazing moment of my then-young life. The smile, the tears, and the joy that exuded from Becky in those immediate seconds spoke volumes about her love for me and for "us." It seemed like she said "yes!" a hundred times. Hugs and kisses came non-stop for the next few minutes—priceless memories in a life that's now so full of them.

It was official. We were engaged. We would be Mr. and Mrs. Paul Wheelock. It seemed the Earth stood still, the planets stopped rotating, and even the sun seemed to shine on this cloudy day as we soaked in that moment.

Eventually we regained our composure, fired up the Buick, and headed for her graduation. We knew we now had a list of things to accomplish before we could wed. First and foremost, we had to get through the graduation, then let our families know of our little secret. We waited until after the ceremony. No point in risking a ruckus before.

At some point during those next couple of hours, her best friend, Teri, saw the ring and understood what had happened. She wasn't too happy about it. Teri thought I had grandstanded— that I was taking away from Becky's special graduation moment.

Becky reaffirmed to me later her excitement, though, and said that Teri would be just fine … and she was.

We shared the news with our families during the meet-and-greet following the ceremony, and thankfully everyone was very happy. I don't think we really surprised anyone other than with the timing.

One of my favorite things to do now is to look at the pictures of Becky sitting with her classmates at graduation and see the smile on her face, lighting up the room. It is a smile that you don't see on a typical graduating-senior's face. The world would go on to see that smile every waking minute of Becky's life for the next 31 years—on days that were perfect and on days when she would struggle to live. A smile that would define who and what she was. A smile that would prove that God was pouring His love through her.

So, it was settled. Becky and I would start the journey that would become our love story, complete with lots of kids, occasional tough times, challenging family situations, and a couple of key battles that would leave us wondering if we had what it took to make it to the end.

The journey would begin with the wedding in April, 1987. The winter couldn't come and go fast enough.

4] THE LION

In the days immediately following the proposal, we spent a lot of time telling everyone we could the good news. We didn't have Facebook or instant messaging or any other social network tools in those days, and so it was a phone call here and a personal visit there. I had already let Mark know that I was going to propose, but I hadn't asked him the obvious question yet. I wanted to do that after it was official and she had said yes. So, I asked Mark to be my best man, and he accepted excitedly and congratulated me profusely.

He was very happy for both of us. Which makes this chapter all that much harder to write?

Christians are familiar with the idea of a battle and how to win one. We are painfully aware that the main purpose of personal battles is to prepare us for the next one ... and the next one. That's not just a Christian thing, of course. Regardless of your faith, think of your own struggles that you've faced, and how they've taught you well ... how they've fortified you for what follows. Personally, I've seen and experienced enough to know that, if I survive one test, another one is waiting for me just around the corner. And it will require every bit of my knowledge, wisdom, strength, and endurance to conquer it.

The title of this chapter is The Lion, illustrated in scripture by young David's battle with Goliath. Everyone likes to focus on David's amazing victory over Goliath ... what a great and courageous battle it was! And yes, it was. But the more important part of the story concerns what David was doing years before he met the giant. He was fighting and winning two smaller battles—with the lion and the bear. I firmly believe, as do theologians, that had David not fought and won those clashes, he would have failed in his bout with Goliath. He wouldn't have had the strength, resolve, courage, or confidence to stand there, sling that stone, and strike his target exactly where necessary. He wouldn't have witnessed God's help. David wouldn't have experienced his faith blossoming—growing with each victory.

This is how it is with us, I believe. God knows our hearts and has seen our lives, beginning to end. He knows what we can handle and when. So, if you think you've been smacked by the ultimate test, the ultimate battle, *The Big One*, and it's going to be all downhill from there, don't celebrate. There's probably a doozy, an even bigger one, on the horizon. Life is a series of getting knocked down and having to get back up. But the more you get knocked down, the harder it will be, each time, to knock you down again. It's called experience and learning.

Our first battle happened in 1986, just eight months before we would exchange our vows. You'll remember that Mark and I had grown apart a bit during 1985 and the first part of 1986. It was bound to happen. He was working, I was working, and when I wasn't working, I was with Becky. Mark and I spent less and less time together but remained great friends. We would talk on the phone, grab a burger in town once in a while, and we would see each other at dances occasionally. I was always there with Becky, and he would often swing in with another friend or two. It was usually great to see him.

One day, in the summer of 1986, Mark met up with us and flashed a smile—the smile that usually lit up the room. Only on this day, the smile seemed different … in fact, everything about him seemed different. He was out of control, bouncing around like he was wired to a lightning bolt, unusually high on energy. We worried that it was drugs.

We didn't know what to say or how to act. This was not the Mark I knew. A few days later, we learned from his mom that he was no longer bouncing off the walls. Now, she said, he was at the other end of the spectrum—deeply depressed. She was very worried and afraid. Something had come over Mark, and none of us had a clue.

Today the term they use for Mark's condition is "bipolar." In those days, it was "manic depressive." Back then, it was difficult to regulate it properly, and the results were often catastrophic. In Mark's case, it would hit him quickly and hit him hard. He would go days with an out-of-this-world high and then—without warning and within minutes, it seemed—he would plummet into the deepest and darkest despair imaginable. His family was shocked and concerned, we were scared and bewildered.

Mark's condition became so bad later that summer that he had to be confined in one of the wards still open at the old Traverse City State Hospital. (The hospital today is no longer a hospital … instead, a friendly, buzzing collection of restaurants, shops, and other tourist attractions. If people could see what went on in those buildings decades ago, I'm not sure the place would be so celebratory.)

I would go visit Mark often, and there were many times he didn't know who I was—or who *he* was. Doctors had put him on medication to level his mood swings, but the level they chose for him was just north of being unconscious. He would sometimes sit and stare with no expression, no awareness.

Occasionally, they would let him leave the facility, and I would take him for a drive around Leelanau County. I would drive for an hour or two, and he would sometimes sit there and never say a word. He'd just stare out the window. Sure, there were times he'd be fairly upbeat, and he would seem to be improving. But that's when the hospital had cut back on the meds; if they didn't get them started again soon, Mark's mood would eventually crash again.

Becky and I had been planning our wedding that summer with great excitement. Meanwhile, I had taken a new job in Traverse City at a production plant working as a spot welder making automotive parts. I'd come home exhausted, frustrated, and doubting I would ever have a job I liked. I was miserable … hating the incredible and debilitating monotony of the work. But it was a job. It was money. On one of those days—actually, a night, since I was then working the 5:30 p.m. to 4 a.m. shift—my manager walked up and said my dad was outside and wanted to talk with me. That was strange. What was my dad doing here at work, at this odd time?

I quickly walked to the parking lot. I could tell immediately from my father's face that something was very wrong, and my first thought was to Becky. Did Becky's dad call my dad about … what?! Before I could ask, my dad spoke the words that would shake my world … launch my first battle … a battle with my own lion.

"Mark is dead," he said.

He had gone home for a visit. He'd been left at the house alone for a bit while his family went out, and feeling frustrated and hopeless, beat up and tired, and wanting this vicious mood cycle to finally be over, he grabbed a favorite shotgun. He loaded it and, in his upstairs bedroom, near a pile of his favorite albums, he placed the barrel to his head and pulled the trigger. It was over. His pain and suffering ended in a blast of anger and confusion.

Later, his brother Jim and I would spend a day trying to clean off those album covers … spots the cleaning company had missed. It's a day I wish I could erase. We sat there cleaning without talking about what we were scrubbing off. We both knew what we were doing; there was nothing more that needed to be said.

Just like that, in that parking lot, my world came crashing down. I remember going home and falling on my bed, crying inconsolably. It would take days to accept that Mark was gone … and how he was gone, and why he was gone. Such tragedy and waste. He had so much to offer. So much life yet to live. How could this gentle, amazingly funny and original guy be gone? How could the closest thing to a brother I would ever know suddenly and violently be no more? All I know is, when I think back on those years, how fortunate and blessed I was to have Becky.

Mark died on September 6, 1986, and Becky and I would be married those eight months later. His brother Jim filled in as best man, and to this day I'm very grateful and blessed that he did. It would take a couple of years into our marriage before the pain of that day would subside … at least enough so I wouldn't break down when I thought of him. Or heard one of his favorite songs. Or handled a shotgun with my dad or granddad. During that time, Becky was my rock—my refuge from the storm. There were many times she would just sit and hold me. No words, no trying to talk it out; she'd just hold me, hug me, love me. Those things saved my life.

This was *our* lion … my first big personal test but also a test of our marriage—our covenant—and our resolve. And we passed the test. We were still alive, still in love, still determined to go on with our lives in spite of the deep pain and sorrow.

As I sit here now and pen these pages, I briefly wonder how I'm supposed to bounce back from the loss of Becky without anyone to hold me, to console me the way Becky did. How can I? Whose bosom am I to tuck into? It's a pain far greater and more unrelenting than what I faced after losing Mark.

But then I realize, of course, that, in this life, struggle is perfect. And I must battle on.

5] THE HONEYMOON MONTHS

What a wedding it was! Some highlights:

First and foremost, my wife to be. Never had I seen such a beautiful and stunning creature as I did that day as she appeared with her dad at the entry to the sanctuary. Again, my heart exploded in my chest, the butterflies went berserk, and every molecule in my DNA couldn't wait to hold her in my arms and kiss her as my bride. I wanted to stop time—to live the scene for as long as I could. I wasn't letting this moment go by without squeezing every good thing I could out of it, and neither was she.

Keith and his wife Robin led the ceremony. What a wonderful job they did—Keith officiating and Robin joining him for a song. They had been married just a short time themselves; their marriage was one that Becky and I looked up to and dreamed we could emulate. Keith was the pastor at Long Lake Friends church, where we started attending when I was a teenager a few years earlier. Little did I know at the time that, decades later, they would officiate a much more powerful and precious moment for us, in that same spot and with many of those same folks in attendance.

We made the mistake of having pictures taken between the wedding and the reception, a horrible and exhausting ordeal. Lots of fake smiles and, eventually, fatigue. All we wanted to do was get to the reception, let our hair down, and begin to celebrate being husband and wife. The reception was a blast; Larry Pleva and the Sound Machine rocked the dance with their usual style and flair. Some of my fondest memories while courting Becky were hanging out with Larry, listening to some of the best music ever, and destroying my hearing one song at a time. No regrets, though. If you can't feel the groove in your chest, then you're not really hearing it. So, what's the point? It was fitting that Larry was there.

A few hours later, we finally arrived at the threshold of our new home. I had purchased the mobile home just a couple weeks earlier. It was on a nice lot in Meadow Lane Village south of Traverse City and was a 1965 vintage. It wasn't much, but it was home.

And now it was late, close to midnight. We were exhausted but still pinching ourselves. We had done it. We were married. I was twenty and Becky was eighteen, and in a few minutes, we were about to embark on an event that would be the first for both of us—a rarity among our peers. It seemed all we heard about from friends or classmates was how someone was "getting some"—on the weekend or at a party or whatever. We were about to do so much more than just "get some." We were about to enter into a level of commitment, trust, and a covenant that God put in the works before we were even conceived. We were about to see and experience each other at one of the most vulnerable and unguarded points in our lives—to engage our souls, our spirit, and our flesh in what scripture describes as, "the two shall become one."

I know that phrase symbolizes more than just sex, but a big part of it does mean the physical consecration of the union. The amazing thing about a moment like this—a moment that you've saved your entire life so that you could share it with just one person—is that it's about so much more. We all know that sex at its basic level is the physical aspect of one body joining another, and all the movement and emotion involved. The result can be euphoria … and maybe a new life. But what we would soon experience was much deeper. We were about to make love with each other's mind, soul, spirit, *and* body. We were about to become one being in the eyes of God. We were about to enter into a level of relationship reserved for those who see themselves as God's children. We were committing to a life of service, sacrifice, and the greatest of all commands, to love God and to love one another as ourselves. We were about to enjoy the most fulfilling moment any couple can enjoy, short of salvation itself.

Just one problem … our intimate encounter was going to have to wait a few more minutes. Some friends had snuck into our mobile home and rearranged our cupboards, messed with the bedding, and did several other cute and fun things to distract us. All it did, though, was intensify the anticipation.

Something else would slow things up a bit, too: the fifty-some buttons that I had to undo, one at a time, up the back of Becky's wedding dress, from her sexy waist all the way to her gorgeous neck. *Dear Lord,* I thought, *I'll never get there!* I can remember that moment like it was yesterday. Every detail of it, even more so now as I sit here alone, pulling up these memories to share with the world. I remember her amazing smell, her perfect and soft hair, and the tingling nerve endings in my hands as I worked each button, slowly making my way from bottom to top.

I'll keep this PG-rated, but my purpose in sharing these details is to convey to those contemplating marriage—and thinking about sleeping with someone prior to marriage—that these are some of the most precious moments you'll ever experience. You only get one take. There are no "do overs." And if you get it right the first time, if you follow the simple rules God has laid out and force yourself to live by the fruits of the spirit, including self-control, then this moment will be just as exhilarating and fulfilling for you as it was for us.

I got to the top button, but instead of unhooking it, I gently touched each side of her beaming face, turning her head so that I could kiss her. We were not new to kissing. But the purity and passion of this kiss would be far beyond anything we'd ever experienced. This kiss would unleash a new level of love and completeness that came directly from God.

I stood, grabbed her hands, and helped her up. Slowly, methodically, with the utmost respect and care, I reached around to the last button, unhooked it, and allowed this incredibly beautiful dress, handmade by her dad's wife Emily, to fall to the floor. Then her other garments followed. I stood there for what seemed like minutes, just staring at her beauty and holding her hands. My heart pounded. There she was in all of her vulnerability, all of her uniqueness, formed perfectly by the creator who knew my needs and wants long before I was born.

She let go of my hands and began a similar process with me—although, I must say, she had it much easier. Six or seven buttons, maybe—a good thing, because by now, anything left on was at risk of being torn off.

What a night that was, some thirty years ago. And what I wouldn't give to experience every detail of it again. I wouldn't change a thing, except maybe to ask Emily to add a few more buttons. Just imagine how much *less* of an experience it would have been had we "gotten some" in the back of a car, or in a bed somewhere?

The next morning we headed to Beulah to stay at the Brookside Inn for a couple of honeymoon days. We would attend a Maynard Ferguson concert at Korson Auditorium in Interlochen, then enjoy an in-room hot tub, a sauna, a steam shower, a mirrored canopy waterbed, and some amazing food. (For the record, we never did go looking to purchase a mirror for our bed at home. That's fun maybe the first or second time, but then it just gets weird.)

We had arrived at "husband and wife." We had consecrated a magnificent union orchestrated by Heaven, and we had settled into our little corner of the world. We were ready and excited to get up each day to see what new adventures, new emotions, and new experiences life had for us.

6] DINNER WITH A TWIST

Shortly after settling into our new used home, we invited a couple over for our first dinner party—the same couple who helped rearrange our home before we arrived on our wedding night. And on the menu: home-made pizza. Dick and Arlene were awesome people; Dick was a groomsman at our wedding. This was our first attempt at making dinner for someone other than ourselves, and oh what fun it was. The preparations began long before they arrived. We cut up the meats and vegetables together. Becky whipped together some dough for the crust. My job was to roll it out and make it nice and round and big enough for the pizza pan.

So, just as I had watched my mom and grandma do a thousand times, I reached for the flour, poured some on the counter, grabbed the rolling pin, and began making my masterpiece. As I rolled and rolled and rolled, I wasn't having much luck with keeping the dough from sticking. I thought Becky must have been off just a bit on one of the dough ingredients. I threw more flour down, then more, and kept rolling. It was a struggle.

After several minutes of a grueling workout, I finally had a crust the size Becky needed for the pan, and off to the assembly line it went. Soon, the pizza was in the oven, the table set, and our guests were on their way. A while later, we were all sitting at the table, hungry. Becky and I were a bit nervous. The pizza looked delicious. We sliced it, served it, said grace, and simultaneously bit into the first dinner for our first guests. Almost in unison and with goofy, mouth-filled "ughs!", the four of us reached the same conclusion: The pizza crust tasted like a sugar cone with meat, cheese, and vegetables on top. I quickly realized what I had done. Yep, I had been grabbing flour out of the wrong canister. Well, not flour. It looked like flour. Felt like flour. But it was powdered sugar. Everyone laughed ... really hard. Dick and Arlene were very gracious, and Becky was so sweet. She was very happy to know she hadn't forgotten something on her end. We skipped the pizza and went right for dessert. We had a lot of fun and good conversation that night.

So, our first meal was a success, sort of. We had a good time with our friends, laughed a lot, and did all of it as husband and wife. We realized that night, and again and again, that we loved just being around each other. We were the very best of friends in every sense of the word. We enjoyed each other's company ... so much so that we had to make deliberate efforts to be with other people like Dick and Arlene. It had been that way since that first cold night in January in Maple City. We didn't need anything or anyone else to complete us or give us purpose. We didn't need alcohol, or clubs, or large parties to feel like we were living life. All we needed was each other, a little nourishment once in a while, and a spot big enough for snuggling, holding hands, and talking about whatever came to mind.

Oh ... and a bed. It's no secret that Becky and I enjoyed our physical relationship. I don't want to share the details. Suffice it to say that making love was a priority multiple times a week and remained that way at least twenty years into our marriage. We loved planning and surprising and teasing and anticipating and romancing each other. Husbands, I will simply say that when you go out of your way to satisfy the senses, the needs, and the emotional wants of your wife, you'll unleash a level of sensuality, desire, and commitment that is unmatched for you on earth.

It was that commitment that became the foundation for our soon-to-expand family.

7] THE GREATEST DECISION EVER

I t was early 1988, and Becky and I were actively talking about starting a family. The conversation centered on whether we wanted to be young parents or old parents. We decided we wanted to start now, so that we'd have many years after they were grown and out of the house to continue our love affair.

We also talked about whether Becky wanted to be a home-maker and a full-time mom, or did she want to work outside the home with a full-time career—or try to do a bit of both? At this point, I had a full-time job with basic benefits doing the spot welding I mentioned earlier; Becky's job was part time with no benefits, working at the gift and ice cream shop at Hilltop Country Corner. Given our expenses, there was no way I could stay home as a house dad. The benefits would be gone, and her income wouldn't be enough. So, if I did that, she would need to find a new full-time job with benefits. If we both wanted to work full time, we would need to pay for day care—expensive!

Neither of us had college degrees or were professionals. And we weren't all that hung up on wealth. That's one of the many things that drew me to Becky in the first place: her practical side and old-fashioned mindset. She loved taking care of me and others. She loved cooking and making a home. She loved being my wife, and the thought of being a mom caused her amazing smile to get even bigger.

So, Becky didn't see that being a homemaker was some kind of slap in the face to womanhood or a degradation of any kind. It was a badge of honor that she could wear with great pride. She felt she could have the most impact on this crazy, screwed-up world by being at home, taking care of whatever kid or kids we'd create.

So, it was decided. We would tweak our finances to fit one paycheck, and we would begin the really fun task of trying to get pregnant. She stopped taking her birth control pills, which made us both happy for a multitude of reasons, including concerns about the safety of the pill.

In early June 1988, Becky shared with me the fantastic news that she was, indeed, pregnant. Her due date was early April 1989. Boy, did the excitement kick in! Becky went from being gorgeous and perfect to stunning and extraordinary over those forty weeks. And her smile seemed to grow right along with her sexy belly.

I also began to appreciate another one of Becky's amazing attributes: her work ethic. I knew she was a hard worker and always incredibly busy. She volunteered in the community. And the fascinating thing was, as she got more and more pregnant and more and more uncomfortable, she didn't slow down or complain. She stayed full speed ahead. She would continue this pattern for five more pregnancies over seven years. She knew only one mode: purposeful joy.

After our first son, Timothy, was born, her doctor looked at her and said, "You have as many babies as you want. Your body is a baby- making machine, and you'll do just fine." I'm not sure he realized what he was unleashing when he spoke those words.

At first, we just wanted two kids. So, Becky eventually was pregnant again. This time, though, we were hoping for a girl— you know, to balance things out. But it was a boy ... another son.

Over time, four more sons would follow as we kept trying for a girl. It just wasn't in the cards. We made boys. That's it. And man, did we make great boys! Six in all, each about seventeen months apart: Timothy, Andrew, David, Stephen, James, and Jonathon, in that order.

But the sixth pregnancy would be our last attempt at a girl. After Jonathon was born, Becky let me know that she wanted to stop.

We didn't want her back on the pill, so we decided that I would go to the doctor for a snip, snip. Only it wasn't exactly snip, snip. I arrived at the doctor's office, nervous, of course. With a needle that seemed much bigger than it was, the doctor began poking me in places where no man ever thought a poke would be helpful or wanted. He needed to numb things up so he could make a small incision, he explained. Incision done, he grabbed the needle again. It looked even bigger than before. He explained that he now needed to numb the vascular ducts so he could clamp them, one at a time, and then snip each to seal them off. Once done, ta-da! No more babies.

The first clamp-snip procedure was easy ... no big deal at all. So, I relaxed a bit and thought this was in the bag, no pun intended. Big mistake ... although, in hindsight, it's good I was relaxed, because I might have kicked the doctor through the wall. He grabbed the clamp, moved over to my left side, and squeezed the clamp tight. Much to my horror—and his shocked surprise—that vascular duct wasn't numb yet. Not even close. So, fellas, imagine the worst kick to the jewels you've ever experienced and multiply it by ten. Holy crap, Batman, did that suck the life out of me.

But we still weren't done. He grabbed the numbing needle and shot me again; he lightly squeezed a bit, but nope, the pain was still there. This went on for about ten minutes ... a shot, then a squeeze ... until he said he couldn't give me any more of the medication because I might never feel anything down there again! He looked a bit perplexed. I told him that sounded just fine, no problem at all, no more shots. "Just do your thing." Finally, and very uncomfortably, he was able to finish.

Home I went and straight to the couch. Becky brought me a bag of frozen peas—the doctor's recommendation—and helped me place it strategically to reduce the swelling. We cuddled on the couch—very non-affectionately, you understand—and had a long movie night. The next day I was on my feet and in full racing form.

8] A LINE IN THE STAIRCASE

During our first year as parents with Tim, and after having drifted away from God, from our church, and from any semblance of holiness in many areas, we found ourselves doing and thinking things we never thought we would.

First, we knew little about raising this first of six sons. He was fussy and wouldn't sleep through the night, but he was also precious and needed us to be the good parents we knew we should be. During that first year, I was also stepping over boundaries I promised to never cross. I started drinking during my two nights a week at league bowling—something Becky detested. Thankfully, I didn't get too carried away with that, although I did drive home drunk after bowling during my twenty-first birthday week. Becky met me at the top of the stairs, which I had just crawled up, and she spoke words that I'd never forget ... and words I'd immediately take to heart. She said she would divorce me sooner than later if this was the lifestyle I planned to lead.

She went on to tell me that she grew up in a family where there was always alcohol—maybe not so much day to day at home, but certainly at all family events and gatherings. She watched family and neighbors sometimes get drunk and obnoxious, and it was something she always hated. She said it was one of the things she adored about me from the start—the fact that I *didn't* drink and never had. My folks didn't drink. My grandparents didn't drink and neither did my uncles, with the exception of the occasional mixed drink at social gatherings. There was never a keg or a refrigerator full of alcohol at the homes of my family, and Becky knew that and loved that. She was looking forward to keeping her home alcohol-free. And here I was bringing it right up the stairs.

This behavior, plus money issues, increased the stress on our marriage shortly after Tim was born. It's also what drove us to a Christian concert at the Lars Hockstead auditorium in Traverse City in the summer of 1990. The group Harvest was playing. There, we both gave our hearts and lives to Jesus, putting aside our own will and desires to begin a journey to recapture the wisdom and understanding that we'd need to raise our children.

We settled into a church during the next couple of weeks; we'd go on to spend fifteen years of our lives there. The drinking stopped immediately. The confidence and wisdom to raise our kids began pouring into each of our hearts, and the kind of love we shared those first few months after we first met came roaring back.

Also adding to the stress, though, was our finances, made worse by our having just one income and my spending habits. I had purchased a really great car we didn't need and a drum set I couldn't afford. I bought a stereo system on credit, plus a fancy television and new VCR. You name it, if we wanted it, I was buying it using easy credit. I, like so many others my age, fell for this false narrative that it was a good thing to have good credit and that if you could use other people's money, why use your own? It was a trap based on idiocy, greed, and impatience.

This would be a battle Becky and I would wage together for years, and something that would cause unnecessary heartache in an otherwise perfect world. And it was completely my fault. But interestingly enough, the hard lessons learned would help us raise, train, and love our kids so they'd become the fine men they are today. They each have a solid understanding of money and how to be good stewards of it. And they also know how easy it is to have fun and live a full life without having, or spending, a lot of money.

There were many weeks during those first few years when I handed Becky twenty-five or thirty dollars for groceries and diapers, because that's all that was left after a car payment, rent payment, gas, and a tithe check to the church. That's when I began to realize what an amazing cook and kitchen genius Becky was. She could grab what seemed a few raw ingredients and, in just a little while, supply the kitchen table with a masterpiece—a meal that would fill our bellies. That talent would continue through six kids ... and after. This woman rocked it, day in and day out, setting a standard that all the boys would long for in their future wives. We had to be frugal then. We had little choice.

I remember one day we had to buy a few groceries and put enough gas in the car to get us to church. But we had no money. Not a cent. It'd be a couple of days until I was paid again. We did have, though, a box in our bedroom where we kept some collectibles, such as coins, savings bonds, and eleven two-dollar bills given to us a few months earlier by a neighbor friend. We grabbed the bills and used half the money to buy some gas and the other half to buy enough food for the two days.

This seemed common during those first ten years, but we never went without, and we always knew God was going to come through somehow, some way. He was very seldom early ... but never late. We always had what we needed, when we needed it. (Although, like the stereo, sometimes what we thought we needed wasn't what we really needed at all.)

Later in our marriage, when we had six sons in tow, we would put together our nickels and treat the family to a dinner at Burger King, Taco House, or the kids' favorite, Pizza Hut. But this was very seldom. It was hard to justify spending on one meal what could have been a week's worth of groceries.

One thing that did seem to happen when we ventured out,

though, was the reception we received from passersby. Numerous people told us how well-behaved and respectful our kids were. We loved that. What Becky didn't love, though, was the occasional comment that, "Your kids are so great and well behaved. *You are so lucky.*" Becky would always tell me later that she just itched to say that luck had nothing to do with it. "Yep, I just dropped these little angels out on the table, and they grew into these perfect little beings, incapable of doing any wrong!" Gosh, that would irritate her.

I'm convinced that most parents grossly underestimate the level of commitment, consistency, and loving discipline necessary to raise responsible, respectful, and decent human beings. What a testament to Becky's desire and her understanding that she was a parent to our children and not a friend. We were charged with raising and equipping them, not shielding and making excuses for them. We were responsible for instilling coping skills, not making sure they were rewarded with a trophy for every attempt at something. We were charged with making sure they were equipped for real life and willing to provide for themselves, not comfortable sitting back and counting on others to do things for them. What a terrific job Becky did all those years, exhausted and overwhelmed at times and very much alone at some points, but always without a word of complaint and never questioning whether I or the kids were worth her efforts. No, she poured her entire being and her entire heart into everything she did, and our sons are the fruit of that success.

One thing Becky and I never did throughout these early years or later in our marriage was to sit around and blame people or events for our predicaments. Most of our problems were self-inflicted. We taught that notion—avoid the blame game—to our sons. We had witnessed too many people playing the victim card. We understood that if we wanted things to be different, we would have to make better decisions. Neither of us needed an MBA to figure that one out.

In fact, this next, major decision would be on us. Totally.

9] THE WORST DECISION EVER

We had been in our little tin-can tube of a home for almost two years when Bud, Becky's dad, pitched an idea to us on the phone. Bud and Becky's mom, Roberta, had recently divorced and were going through the agonizing aftereffects. Bud and his new wife Emily had bought some property in Michigan's Upper Peninsula and were moving there. (Becky was devastated that he was moving out of town at a time when our babies—his grandkids—were being born and our family was just getting started. She cried many times over that situation.) As a way for Bud to help settle up with Becky's mom, he and the credit union manager, Bob, proposed that Becky and I buy the house using an assumed-mortgage plan. So, Bud would unload this burden, but we would get a bigger house.

Yes, we were looking to move at some point into something bigger. We had one child, Tim, and were talking about a second. I was grossing $240 a week. Becky was at home being a mom and homemaker. We already had a $150-a-month car payment. But the credit union manager and Bud convinced us that we could afford a $515-a-month house payment.

We should have never taken that phone call. It was the single, worst decision we would make in our married life. It would send us spiraling out of control financially for years.

There was one plus, though: The house was next door to Becky's Grandma Boone. She was the one shining star in the midst of our financial black hole, and she helped where she could. How Becky loved to sit and visit with her. They would can together, snip beans together, take walks together, and play with Tim and eventually Andy together. A favorite memory of Becky's was of Grandma Boone feeding our boys cheese puffs with a toothpick like birds, one at a time, so they wouldn't get their hands dirty and subsequently, her kitchen. Those were fantastic days and great memories.

But we couldn't make the finances work. So, we had to eventually sell the house. It devastated us and Grandma Boone both. At one point, while waiting for it to sell, we got 90 days behind on our house payments. It ruined our credit score for years.

Needless to say, those were some tough months, and Becky did all she could to maintain a level of respect for her dad and stay in touch with him. The combination of him leaving and not being a major part of her sons' lives, and the financial stress of buying a house and having it only benefit her divorcing parents, was crushing.

We finally sold the house in late 1991 and headed for our third move as husband and wife. But it would be years before we could afford our own home. Buying that house was a decision that I would regret for years. It happened because we were too eager to have what our parents had, or at least what we thought was important that they had. It was a decision that would make me angry and embarrassed because of my inability to fix it. Becky, too, felt bad because she thought she wasn't contributing by earning a paycheck. I would always reassure her that she was the one working the hardest, and that what she was doing at home with the kids would ultimately get this family out of a hole and into something great.

I didn't know then, of course, that we would eventually own our own business, and—better yet—that all of our kids would eventually have roles in the success of that enterprise. They would end up being the very best fruit of Becky's diligent work at home as a mom.

In hindsight, this experience was just one of many that would strengthen our marriage, our bond and our resolve. And thankfully, it would also strengthen all those relationships years later, when it really mattered and when we had the wisdom and insight to see the bigger picture.

As we moved from place to place, we gathered memories. Here's one: We had rented an upstairs apartment from an elderly woman in Traverse City. One winter's day, I arrived home from a Saturday Bible school downstate that I regularly attended with a few guys from our church. I walked upstairs to hear David, son number three and only a month or two old, fussing like crazy. He'd been doing this consistently for a couple of weeks now, and we were concerned about his health and about ready to have him checked out.

As I reached the top of the stairs, I was met with 84-degree air. It was like a sauna. And then I realized the problem: Our land lady downstairs was always cold. The house had very little insulation, and so she would run the furnace hard during the winter months. Most of the heat would rise right into our apartment. I looked over at David, who was fussing like crazy, and the light bulb went off. He was dressed in a diaper and onesie and was in his combination car seat/rocking chair, covered with a light blanket. I walked across the room, knelt down, removed the blanket, took off the onesie, and laid him on a blanket outside the seat in just his diaper.

If looks could write a book, that kid wrote a novel entitled, "Thank You." With one deep, precious sigh, he relaxed, stopped fussing, and turned into the cutest and most-contented baby ever. To this day, David sleeps with a fan on and very few blankets. The guy's a walking heat lamp. I was a hero with Becky that day.

After being in the apartment just seven months, in 1992, we moved to another apartment above Hilltop Country Corners at

Hilltop Road and M-22, not too far from where Becky grew up and I proposed. This proved to be a great place to live for almost two years, because Becky could work part-time in the craft store and ice cream shop while still raising our babies. A friend of ours babysat Tim, Andy, and David from time to time, and this is where our son Stephen would call his first home. Becky had worked there the first two years of our marriage, and she was thrilled to be back. We loved the owner, Kay, who had lost her husband, Bob, to cancer in 1989, a week after Tim was born.

It also is where we lived when I took the worst job of my entire life—a job I would hold for only four months in early 1993.

I had worked for a heating-and-cooling-equipment whole-saler since 1989 and wasn't going anywhere financially. Don, a great friend from church, mentioned that the bread-vending company he worked for was hiring. Good money, great benefits, and a secure future, he said. So, I was hired. Soon I was up at 3 a.m. each day. As the new guy, though, I had the worst route with the least revenue. That was only fair and wasn't a problem. What was a problem was I was usually running behind in my route by 5 a.m. So, I'd end up working sometimes fourteen hours a day for just three or four hundred dollars a week. I'd come home completely exhausted. With a new baby at home and absolutely nothing left for him or my wife, I was toast—and the stress was killing me.

I called Becky from a pay phone in Frankfort one day and told her I was leaving the truck there and walking home. I was done. I was emotionally spent at every level. Becky, speaking softly and acknowledging my pain, told me I couldn't do that because that's not who I was, and I would regret it. She convinced me to finish my day and to come home, and she would take care of me. Together, she said, we would make the decision to move on and try something else.

I had never loved her more than I did that day. She was my hero, my security, and my reward, all in the same afternoon. She didn't care a bit about the money and cared in every way about my wellbeing. What an incredible woman.

We would stay at Hilltop a couple of years, enjoy ice cream in homemade waffle cones on the front porch swing, watch the bay in the evenings, and dream about owning our own home. We thought we were in heaven and living the dream. A covered front porch, a view of the bay, and all the ice cream we could eat.

We eventually knew we'd need another place to live, though, because Kay was making different plans for the business and the apartment. Plus, we really wanted something more permanent. We didn't have money for a down payment, and we didn't own any land. We weren't going to afford a home on property anywhere in Leelanau at the time, and so we again began looking at mobile homes. Only this time, we were going to buy our own— something new and much nicer. It was a 1994 model complete with a shingled roof, eaves, vinyl siding, and thermopane windows. It was 1,280 square feet with three bedrooms and two full baths and was energy efficient to the core.

What a great home it was. The only problem was that we had to park it on a rented lot at the back of the mobile-home park, and the lot rent combined with the house payment would almost eat us alive for three years.

Limping along financially, we decided, again, that we had to make a change. We placed a for-sale sign in the window and began to advertise a little. It was a quality home in very good condition, and we were confident we'd get it sold. But after almost a year on the market, our confidence shrank. Then, on a Saturday morning in March, the phone rang. A lady from Kingsley asked if she could come by and see the place in about twenty minutes, and we agreed. She stepped into the house, walked to the end with the master bedroom first, then walked to the other end and back to the door. She took only five minutes to look around, said she liked it and she'd be in touch, then left.

Two days later, on Monday morning, the bank called to verify a few things. A couple of hours later, we had a full-price offer, paperwork to sign, and thirty days to get out. "Now what?!" we asked each other. We had to pack, find another home, and move out in thirty days. We were in high gear once again.

It would take almost the full thirty days to find a place. Because it was early in 1997, we found a vacant seasonal rental where we could stay for two months. But we had to move all of our stuff into a garage and leave it packed up and continue searching for a more permanent home. The rental was neat, though, because it was directly across the street from the church where we were married—and from Keith and Robin, the pastor and his wife who married us.

It would take almost the entire sixty days to find something, and what we found would end up being the place our boys would love and where so many incredible memories would be made.

It was an old farmhouse at the Golden Valley Ranch near the nearby, small town of Empire, and the rent was finally something we could afford. We moved in the summer of 1997 and stayed there five years, the longest stretch so far and the sixth place we called home in our ten-year marriage.

It was in this house that Becky would fully implement home-schooling our sons. It's where Tim would fall through a rotted, wooden sewer cover, James would take a dump in the front yard during a horse show complete with spectators, and I would step into the shower one morning and get electrocuted while touching the wall and the soap tray at the same time.

On the first night there, we were able to see stars in all their detail for the first time in our marriage. The moon was just bright enough that we could see each other. And there was no sound of neighbors as far as we could hear.

It was also the home where we would own our first computer, gather our own firewood for heat all winter long, and replace about every window because of a flying shoe, golf balls, and toys. It's the home where Becky and I would sleep on just a mattress because our box spring wouldn't fit up the tight staircase, and it's the home where Becky, much to her horror, learned that mice climb stairs and cats bring them to bed with you.

It's also the home where we would have our first pet dog. Up until then, it had been just cats. In the fall of 1997, on Becky's birthday, September 12, I surprised her and the kids with our greatest pet to date, a Golden Retriever, Autumn. She was just nine weeks old when I carried her in and laid her on Becky's lap. I was the hero once again. All seven in the family thought I was king.

This is also where we were living the morning I got a phone call from Becky on one of our first cell phones letting me know that she had rolled our mini-van but everyone was okay. The van was totaled and upside down, but there was not a scratch on anyone. That day, we were incredibly thankful to God for His protection and mercy.

What a place. We would help treat trauma wounds to horses, help a girl with a broken back who fell off one of those horses, spend hours playing in the snow with the ranch tractor, and play in the mud on our mountain bikes in the front yard. All six boys bunked in the same room, and they learned to write sentences there and appreciate what it meant to love their brothers and figure out how to settle things without mom's help.

We were just five minutes to the Empire beach, seven minutes to Glen Arbor, ten minutes to relatives, and directly across the street from inexpensive and often free golf at the Dunes. The people working there knew our sons by voice when they called out. That was cool.

This was also the home where we would master the "staycation." This house would allow us to save some money and actually start to think it possible to purchase our own, stick-built house. But only if we could put a little money aside.

So, we stayed home, climbed trees, played basketball in the backyard, went mountain biking, and spent countless hours at the beach, all on a few pennies worth of gas most days. It was where Becky and I learned to be frugal by choice rather than necessity, and where we were beginning to mature in our decision-making process.

This would be the launching place for our new lives as homeowners, business owners, public-school attendees, and fans of countless basketball games, including a state championship game some eight years later in 2010. This was the home that really started it all for our family. We had come a long way since we'd made that financial blunder of buying Becky's parents' home. Looking back, each move was a stepping stone to get where we needed to be now. We were done overreaching financially ... done being naive. We were finally on track, and life was wonderful.

10]   A PARTING OF THE WAY

One thing constant in our lives since 1990 was our attendance at a church in the middle of Leelanau County. We attended service there three times a week—Sunday morning and evening and Wednesday nights. I won't spend a lot of time recalling our fifteen years there. I could write another book just on our journey through that long and often painful experience. I do need to mention some highlights, though.

The church was the best and worst thing that ever happened to our family. The messages were awesome. The teaching, the challenges to live holy, the lessons learned, and the nuggets taken away to help live everyday life were priceless. But along the way we allowed the pervasive, critical attitudes of so many to wear off on us. We began thinking too highly of ourselves. We alienated our families for years. We missed out on birthday parties, weddings, graduations, Super Bowl parties, and the like because we were in church leadership, and we had to attend church or be chastised by members the next time we showed up.

We began to think we were the cream of the crop in the Christian world. We thought we had all the right answers for everyone else, and we fully believed that God wanted us to be in church whenever the doors were open. We did that at tremendous financial cost to our family. I couldn't work a second or third job or work overtime because I believed that if I walked in faith, attended church, and trusted God, He would provide. We also inflicted horrible relational costs on our parents, siblings, and close friends.

Finally, after fifteen years of sitting in leadership meetings where we ganged up on others who had left our tight circle, I had reached my limit. I was being given the usual "trust God and have faith and your financial needs will be met" spiel by the same guy who always preached it to me. I looked him in the eye and simply said that if he or the church or anyone in the church would like to start writing me checks to pay my bills, I'd be happy to be at church seven days a week, 'round the clock, willing and able to do anything they needed.

But until then, I said, I was going to start earning more income as God blesses me to do so—and begin living life on planet Earth among normal, realistic people.

What made it worse was how we'd come to this discussion. I had been listening to this man, a church member who had mentored me for years and led me to Christ in a deep and fantastic way. He sat across the table and told me that he had just recently stopped and visited another former leader of the church—a good friend of Becky's and mine—and that all this guy did was talk about work and money and worldly stuff and nothing about God or Jesus or church or anything.

It just so happened that I had actually been at this man's place of business the week prior and had asked specifically if he had talked with any of the other members of the leadership team lately. He said he hadn't seen anyone in ages, and definitely hadn't seen the gentleman who was telling me the story across the table in more than two years.

In short, my mentor was lying to me. So that was the final leadership meeting I would attend. Later, after Becky and I had a chance to go for a walk and discuss the concerns we'd both been having, we decided to part ways with that ministry. Within seconds of that decision, a weight lifted off our shoulders, and the winds blew fresh in our faces. For the first time in years, we felt free. We could actually begin to live our lives for God and for each other.

If I allow myself to ponder all the hundreds of hours I spent away from Becky doing "church" stuff, or with Becky but focused on other "church" things, I feel regretful and angry. So, I just don't go there. In the end, we didn't leave with a lot of fanfare. There were no arguments or drama of any kind. We simply resigned our positions and faded away. To this day, there has never been a conversation as to why we left.

Thankfully, today, there are no hard feelings. Some of our dearest friends still attend and pastor there. (The church would prove monumental in pulling off the feeding of almost 400 people the day of Becky's memorial service.) And there were no hard feelings then. Just the somber and experiential caution as we moved forward, loving God, living according to what we had learned, and looking to see if there was any other church that we could call home. That would prove quite the chore.

11]   A SENSUAL BREEZE, A BED UNDEFILED

Thilere are a million things that can make a marriage magnificent. But only a few are necessary to destroy one quickly and completely. At the top of that list, of course, is the decision to share a bed and body with another person outside of that covenant. Suffice it to say, we didn't roll that way.

What follows next is my attempt to convey in an open way what made our story so incredibly special and long-lasting, and fortified us for the future. I'll be sharing some private details here. Why? Because I believe Becky and I were living a romance blessed by God, unshakeable, and one for the ages. It was a kind of marriage unfamiliar to many within our own families, on both sides; it would eventually hold us strong and unshakeable in the face of a brutal and unrelenting enemy, Becky's cancer.

Early in our walk with God, we learned that He was the one who made our marriage bed what it was. He would be the one to give us the desires and the means to satisfy those desires. We knew that as long as we were faithful to one another and used those intimate moments to honor Him, we really couldn't go wrong. Creativity and spontaneity would be a blessing from God and would help keep the fires lit for decades.

One such moment—and even now, it gives me goosebumps—happened on the first night we moved into our Empire home, in the summer of 1997. Up until then, for all of our marriage, we were surrounded by neighbors on all sides, below, and even above. The Empire house at night was quiet and secluded. So, after the horse activities settled down on the ranch, and our kids were settled into bed, Becky and I had seventy acres and deep darkness to explore.

You may recall how Becky and I could see brightly lit stars on that first night at the Empire house. Well, we saw those from atop a very sturdy and handily convenient picnic table left there by the previous tenants. As we sat on that table, holding each other and staring at a celestial picture we hadn't seen in years, the romance of the moment got to us. This was the first time we had made love outside; it would not be the last.

Such outdoors intimacy didn't just happen in our acreage. One of the things that Becky and I loved to do was take the kids over to the beach at Port Oneida for swimming. They loved the big waves, and our Golden Retriever loved swimming there for hours. During most summer nights and weekends, the family could be found on either that beach or the beach in Empire. What was great about the Port Oneida beach, though, was its solitude. The family often had the whole shoreline to ourselves.

Beginning in 2006, when Becky and I became self-employed, we started a marriage tradition just for the two of us. No kids, no friends, no family; nobody. On the first day the temperature hit 80 degrees, we would record a voicemail message saying the office was closed for the afternoon. Then we'd pack a beach blanket, a camera for the sunset, a bucket for rocks, a towel or two for our wet feet, our favorite cologne and perfume, and some very comfy and easily removed articles of clothing. We'd jump in the car and head for Port Oneida.

I can still remember that first year. Then, the water level was relatively low, so there was an endless beach and lots of coves. It was easy to find privacy. We had completed our rock hunting, walking back and forth along the beach. After bumping into one another, stopping for the occasional kiss, hug, and caressing of a hand, the moment came to enjoy each other just as we did on that picnic table years earlier.

And again, God did not disappoint. A gorgeous sunset, a warm breeze, and the sound of crashing waves, seagulls, and tall grasses swaying proved the perfect setting.

During the long, winter months that followed, we would find ourselves hinting to each other about spring being just around the corner. We'd wonder how many more days were left until the thermometer hit 80. Over time, this little oasis on the sand became heaven on earth for us—even during those years when I had to help carry Becky up and down the trail to the beach because she was too weak to do it on her own.

This tradition would prove one of the most painful to lose. Just days after losing Becky, the temperature turned 80.

It was through moments like this, though, that we saw our relationship deepen and our ability to be tempted by anything or anyone else thwarted. That romance and spontaneity helped forge an environment that our kids would intuitively recognize as an awesome and loving relationship; they knew we were best friends and mutual caregivers. It was a level of intimacy and devotion that we had never seen on TV, heard about in the movies, or read about in any books.

Two other examples, and then we'll move on.

First, there was the spring of our seventeenth wedding anniversary in 2004. Becky's life was full of nonstop care of myself and the boys, and she worked tirelessly as a homemaker, mother, and wife, and even helped at the kids' school. This incredible woman, who rarely complained, worked a million times harder than any of the seven of us.

Becky would always keep a list of gift suggestions for herself on the fridge, so that each of the boys could find ideas for her birthday and Mother's Day. The boys thought this was pretty funny ... always worth a chuckle. You might think Becky was being kind of selfish, but she did this to instill in our sons the importance of being good husbands—so that when they became husbands, they would cherish such dates as a time to give back to their wives.

What she didn't know was that by doing this, she was also reminding *me* of my responsibility to cherish her!

So that spring, I knew that Becky needed a break, and I needed to give that to her. It had to be stress-free for her ... totally pre-planned. A surprise. I wanted to sweep her off her feet just like I did on our wedding night and pretend for just a little while that it was just her and me again. No other responsibilities. Just loving, laughing, and reenergizing.

I decided she needed a long weekend away. But I had to start weeks in advance to plan it out. You don't easily find sitters for six kids, especially if you're keeping it a surprise for supermom.

I created the perfect plan. Earlier, I had been doing some sales calls—trying to sell Christmas lighting—and one of the places I visited was a resort near Acme. While there, the manager agreed to let me see one of their high-end suites overlooking the bay. Wow. It was amazing in size, complete with a separate living room, a Jacuzzi spa tub, a fireplace, and fantastic views out two different sides of the room.

Keep in mind that money was still very tight, and what I was considering spending for two nights and three days at this place would buy groceries for a month. The money wasn't an issue, really. I just wanted to make sure that if I was going to spend it, the weekend would be perfect in every detail.

I arranged things with the manager, and he agreed to be part of the plan. Before the time came, I packed the kids' bags and got them to the appropriate sitters; the boys were not all staying with the same family. They would go to their respective spots after school.

Then the big day arrived. I told Becky I was going to make a couple of sales calls and really wanted her to go with me—just so we could spend a few extra hours together. Since the kids were in school, she agreed. I had already had our bags delivered to the suite, brought flowers in and put them on display, picked up some of her favorite chocolates, and even bought her some new lingerie just for this occasion. We arrived at the resort, and I asked her to come in so she could see how beautiful it was. I also asked her if she'd ever thought of staying at such a place. She just smiled.

We met the manager, and I asked if he had a minute to show us one of those fancy rooms. He smiled, said "Sure!" and led us to the suite I had reserved. He opened the door, and I let Becky step in first, holding her hand while I followed behind her.

It took a minute for her to see the flowers and our luggage bags. And then the tears began falling. She turned and jumped into my arms. The manager quietly dismissed himself, and Becky and I went on to have a powerful couple of nights, laughing, snuggling, watching a favorite movie or two … and much more.

And now the final example. In the year 2000, I turned into a truck driver, steering a semi-truck all over the country. Becky on occasion would come along for the ride. Becky loved riding with me, and she loved the stories I would tell. Like the one about the lady who flashed her boobs at me as she drove by. Or the young black woman in Texas who woke me up early one morning and wanted to know if I wanted some brown sugar for breakfast. (After clearing my head, I rolled down the window and replied, "No thanks, sweetheart; I've got all the white sugar I need at home.") One thing I always did was call Becky right away when these kind of things happened, both to make her laugh and to help reassure her that I was hers and hers only. She had given her entire life to our marriage to that point, and it wasn't lost on me.

So, events like these, and the weirdness of the back-and-forth conversations on the CB radio, gave Becky an inkling of the trucker life.

One of the trips with Becky was to upstate New York. We found sitters for all the kids, loaded the trailer, and headed east.

It would only be a four-day trip. We eventually dropped our outbound load, then headed for Buffalo for one of two pickups that would get us back to Michigan. This trip would be full of surprises. For instance, we needed a guy to stand on top of a junkyard car, watching to make sure we cleared a low bridge—a problem caused when I made a wrong turn in urban Buffalo. Then there was the sight of the adorable family of Amish kids walking home from school in the back country of New York, where we made our second stop on the way home ... to pick up goat cheese near their farm.

We would stop at truck stops for a shower, a fresh set of clothes, and dinner. I'd walk into the truck stop holding Becky's hand, or have my arm wrapped around her shoulder or waist. It made my day when the room full of other truckers—men just like me—would stare. I knew what they were thinking: "Man, would you look at that lucky S.O.B." "She's gorgeous." "What is she doing with him?"

I know it might seem strange, but I felt like the luckiest and most blessed husband on the planet when I walked through a room like that. I beamed with pride and thanked God that she was mine and that my world was perfect because of her.

We got to Detroit, unloaded and fully expected to be routed back to Traverse City with an empty trailer. God had other plans. Instead, we were routed to Sandusky, Ohio, to pick up roofing shingles. We weren't happy about the delay. We needed to get home, free our babysitters, and get Becky back to her usual element.

I was familiar with this stop and what we might be facing: a long line of trucks and a long dock time getting the trailer loaded. But during the two-hour ride to Sandusky, we began to look at the brighter side of things; God began working on our hearts. By the time we arrived, we had completely turned our attitudes around. We were now hoping for a long wait time so we could hang out in the truck together and relax.

We arrived and were told we would be getting a dock but it

would be close to six or seven hours before we would be loaded. The dock guy thought for sure we'd be upset. We just smiled and said thanks. We opened the trailer doors, backed in the truck, and parked.

We had some food with us, so we started by eating and listening to some music. Then, after a while, we retired to the bunk. One of the trucks I drove had an actual table in it, but this truck cab had a set of bunk beds; we had the top bunk flipped up.

Becky sat with her back against the back of the bunk wall, and I laid my head in her lap. Now bear with me on the details that follow. I'm going to tell you more than you probably want to know, but there's a reason. We began to undress each other but just from the waist up. As I settled my head into her chest, and her arms lay across mine, there was hardly anything sexual about it. And that was a new experience for us ... an unfamiliar sensation.

We began to talk about things at a depth we'd not done before as husband and wife. Remember my drinking problems, the family divorces, and Mark's death? This is the day when I would begin to bear my soul to Becky ... share stories from my youth about things I'd never told ... things too personal and painful for this book. I would ask for forgiveness from her, and I would pledge my undying love and devotion. She shared similar things with me, and we talked about what we thought our marriage could be.

Over the next four hours, we laid there and talked, cried, held each other tight in reassurance, and communicated at a level neither of us knew was even possible. No sex, no foreplay, just a closeness and a connection that to this day is void of words to explain and more powerful than my brain can put into terms.

It was a spiritual moment brought by God. We would kiss, caress, hug, cry, shake, tremble, and pray together. Eventually, as we grew closer and more intimate in our conversation, and as our connection grew deeper than ever before, we made love. But this was so different for us. We were, quite literally, making love to each other's mind, will, and emotions, as well as body. We were engaged at the deepest levels of intimacy, and every breath, every movement, every word, and every thought were as if we were sharing one body, one heart, one spirit. It was ten times more powerful and intimate than even our wedding night.

I often think of that day since Becky's passing and hope that when I meet her again, we can again experience the depth of that oneness ... and that it lasts for eternity.

We eventually felt the fork truck start placing pallets aboard the trailer, and about an hour later we were headed home. Over those next several weeks, more than a few people asked why we had such a glow about us, why we were sooooo happy, and what was our secret to being that way. Just like now, we couldn't find the exact words to describe it. All we could say was that we were madly, deeply, and completely in love, and that God was the very center of it all in a profound and eternal way.

These are the memories that sustain me now in my darkest of days. They are the memories that make me long for Heaven, for Jesus, and for Becky like never before. And they are the memories I want to share with my family, our sons, and the world in hopes that others will make a deliberate effort to ask God to turn their marriage into an epic and amazing love story of their own.

12) ADVENTURES AND MISADVENTURES

A few years before we began the Port Oneida adventures, we used to go camping with the kids. One of our favorite places to go for a late-summer or early-fall weekend was to the Pigeon River State Forest Campground, just north of the tiny berg of Vanderbilt. We loved going there because we had gotten into mountain biking with the older kids. So, with the fifteen miles of those trails near the campground, the eighty-plus miles of hiking trails, and the campground being right on the river, there was plenty for all of us to do. We had no cell phones, no pagers, no music devices, and no TV … just a couple of tents, some great food, and a fire for telling lots of stories and creating laughs with the kids—memories that we share to this day.

Here are just a few of those memories:

Jonathon was fairly young, about four, and had just learned how to ride his mountain bike. Scattered on the edge of our campsite were those short, round, brown, pine poles often used to separate campsites. Jonny was attempting some trick on his bike when he lost control while going pretty fast. His front tire slammed head on against one of those poles. The bike abruptly stopped, but Jonny didn't. He flew forward, smashing his family jewels against the handlebar support. He then fell flat atop the pine pole—and smashed the jewels again. With only about twenty inches to go before hitting the ground, he twisted over to his back, slid off the pine pole, hit the ground with a "plop," and let out a cry … only to have the teetering bike land squarely—yep—on the family jewels.

Three painful strikes in just two and a half seconds. A mountain of trouble from a mountain bike. I hate to say it now, but his cries of pain were quickly drowned out by laughter from the family.

Later that same night, James thought it would be funny to stick his bare butt in Jonny's face while the six boys were getting ready for bed in their own big tent. Becky and I were sitting by the fire and heard the commotion.

Then I had an idea. A disturbing idea, sure. But a perfect payback on behalf of Jonny. I walked to the tent, dropped my drawers just below my butt cheeks, and bent over with my hiney up against the opening of the tent. I yelled to the kids that there was something very cool to see "in the full moon." There was, in fact, a full moon that night. Then I yelled to James to open the tent so everyone could see.

James unzipped the screen door and poked his face out … and saw the most unsettling full moon ever. The eight of us chuckled about the payback well into the night, and James forever thought twice about pranking his brothers.

On another trip, my dad and I gathered up our bikes and our three oldest—Timothy, Andrew, and David—and headed for Pigeon River for another weekend of camping and riding. During these trips, we really enjoyed treating ourselves to tasty food over a fire and lots of snacks—the latter not the norm at home. So, after biking all day, we started a fire and cooked chicken-alfredo packets, seasoned chicken breasts, and some veggies. After dinner, we shared lots of snacks, red fruit punch, pop, and a host of other things. The boys were in food heaven … for a while, anyway. They would soon find themselves in outhouse hell. Not used to eating that much nor eating such rich items, each of the three boys would spend most of the night racing to the outhouse and back.

At one point, David didn't wake up in time and left a rank reminder of the night's snacks on my sleeping bag while rushing out the door. It was a mix of interesting sounds—projectile liquid shooting from his nether regions and his groans all the way up the walk.

I shouldn't have been surprised, though. David had a reputation for this kind of thing. Several years earlier, while ushering the kids out to the car where Becky was waiting to ride to church, I noticed that David was missing. I headed back into our mobile home, and as I walked down the hallway, a scary odor smacked me in the nostrils. In a very concerned yet apprehensive tone, I asked David where he was and if he was all right. He answered quietly that he was in the bathroom and needed some help.

I opened the door and there was David with his pants down—and liquid diarrhea on the wall, the toilet, the floor, the vanity, the other wall, the base of the tub, and the toilet paper roll. It was like someone made him bend over, ordered him to squeeze as hard as he could from inside, then spun him like a top.

I was usually the parent who handled the blood and broken things; Becky was usually the parent who handled the poop and vomit. So, I told David not to move, went outside to Becky, told her David "had an issue," then sat in the front seat waiting to hear, "Oh My God!"

I'm pretty sure we skipped church that day.

That night in the campground was a bit like that. And the next day, the three boys looked rumpled and worn out … like they'd been dragged through a knothole. My dad and I proceeded to eat most of the rest of the food. No one else seemed hungry.

13]   A DREAM FINALLY REALIZED

W hat a blast we had in Empire. So many great memories with the kids, new jobs that allowed me to be home every day and, finally, the daylight at the end of the tunnel we had been working so hard to see. After years of struggling financially, most of it self-inflicted, we were finally talking seriously about being first time-home buyers. And yes, I say first time, because this would be the first time that we, alone, based on our own finances, wisdom, and experience, would be purchasing a home. Oh, how I wished we could have started over in 1989 and made better decisions. But those eggs can never be unscrambled. We were moving on—and about to realize a big dream.

There is one last thing that happened in Empire, though, that needs telling. I realize now that this was the hint of the cycle of trials, hardships, battles with self-esteem, and medical issues that Becky would face for fourteen years to come. The irony is that it started at the very same time we felt so uplifted about our lives and future.

If I were to pull out a couple of pictures of Becky during our stay at the Empire house, you'd immediately see the problem. At the time, we hadn't really noticed, because it was such a gradual change. Becky had started to put on weight, retain lots of fluids—most notably in her face and eyes—and she was consistently very tired. She slept often, had little energy or motivation while awake, and just plain seemed worn out mentally most of the time. It was the fatigue and sleeping that finally got our attention, and it warranted a visit to her doctor.

Tests revealed an almost nonfunctioning thyroid. One of the docs said in amazement that most people in Becky's condition would be in a very deep sleep around the clock, if not in a full-blown coma. According to her medical team, she was very fortunate to not have suffered any long-term effects. Following a few lab draws and consults with her doctor, Becky got the medicine she needed, and within a few days, she was back to her old, energetic self. What a happy girl she was.

We had contacted our bank about the possibility of a home loan, and the loan officer there gave us a number and the green light to go house shopping. You can't imagine our joy. Finally, after years of living paycheck to paycheck, and still going backwards, we were about to become home owners—with our own garden, our own well, our own grass, our own neighbors, our own garage, and our own mortgage payment. It took some time to find a home in our price range in Leelanau County, where we really wanted to be, but with persistence, a little luck, and God knowing our hearts' desires, we found a small, three-bedroom ranch house with a one-car garage on a half-acre in Elmwood Township, just inside the county line. It was close to Traverse City, close to family, and the closest we had ever been to our church.

We moved in on October 12, 2002, a full month after the kids had started attending Suttons Bay schools. Becky had been driving them up there every day from Empire. We filled up that ranch in short order. It was easy to heat, easy on electricity, and virtually maintenance free. And my sweetheart had her own kitchen and her own dining room where she would spend the next twelve years enriching the lives of all of us—our friends, our kids' friends, our families, and our neighbors. She would host Thanksgiving dinners, cookie decorating parties, birthday parties, and a bunch of other events in that room, and she would fill it with her radiant smile—even on days when there was not much to smile about.

The house was ours, and Becky magnificently turned it into a home. It became the final stepping stone for our sons as they marched to adulthood ... the place where so many of their ideas and aspirations started. We planned to live here forever. We knew that as the kids left, one by one, the house would get bigger, and we'd have more room. So why, ever, look for a different house? After fifteen years of marriage, bringing six sons into the world, and living in seven other homes, we had finally settled.

Just a couple of months after moving in, I started working for a downstate pest control company that had acquired a local business. Up until then, I had worked in the wholesale heating and air conditioning business ... for almost twelve years ... then drove trucks all over the country, then came back to the heating/air conditioning job, and eventually moved into HVAC contracting. Just a week after starting the latter job, though, terrorists collapsed the twin towers of the World Trade Center, and commercial spending declined steeply. My new boss, a very gracious and honest man, gave me a six-month notice that he'd have to let me go because business was way off. It was also a job that was quite a bit out of my league, and he and I both knew in an unspoken way that I probably didn't have much of a future there. I appreciate to this day the opportunity Dan gave me and the way in which he let me go. Dan is a good man, and my family will be forever grateful. He also loved, loved, loved Becky's homemade pies.

So, I jumped back in a truck for a couple of months while waiting for the pest control gig to open up, and when it did, off I went. I spent a couple of weeks downstate in manager training, since I would be running the operation. Becky would later come on board as our customer service representative. We would get to work together, all day, every day. We had never done that before, and we knew that for many couples, it can prove to be their undoing. But not us. Just like in marriage, it was a match made in Heaven.

I just wish the company we worked for was as good a match. In a nutshell, this Detroit company was never happy and always wanted more—more hours from its staff and more profits for its shareholders. In the first year, Becky was putting in full-time hours when she had only agreed to work part time. I was getting paid for forty hours a week but was working a minimum of seventy-five to eighty hours. Then, my well-deserved bonus was eliminated because another branch hadn't performed well. That was the breaking point. We decided to resign. Our marriage was suffering, our kids were suffering, and our personal-life goals and desires were suffering.

We left in the summer of 2005 after giving our two weeks' notice. As we looked back, we wished we had just walked out the door and never again spoken a word to those arrogant and predatory people. We needed an income, obviously, and we needed to pay for this house we had bought three years prior, and so I went back to work driving a truck. It was something I knew how to do, I could make decent money at it, and the trucking company would work to get me home more often than not. We actually began discussing buying our own truck and me driving full time as an owner-operator.

We wrestled with that decision until mid-winter and then decided on another path, a path that would be wrought with heartache, challenges, vipers, snakes, and pride. It would ultimately allow us to realize more dreams than we ever dared imagine. It would allow us to fight a battle that we would ultimately lose, but be able to fight side by side, every inch of the way, all day, every day. And that would prove to be priceless, and a blessing from God Himself.

14]   THE BEAR

E very job we ever had required that we punch a clock or fill out a time sheet. So, we worked a set number of hours for a set wage. Once in a while, though, employers can take advantage of you—if you let them. That was the case with the pest control company. I figured that Becky and I were working an average of less than $8 an hour for the company. We were more than eager to say adios.

As I drove around the country in a new Peterbilt tractor, though, Becky and I would talk over the cell phone about the future. We didn't see the trucking job as a permanent one. During the winter of 2005/2006, we decided on another route: Since I was still a licensed, commercial pest-control applicator with over two years' experience—and so would qualify for the business license—why not bet on ourselves? So that's what we did. We started our own company.

I made the mistake, though, of taking legal counsel from an accountant who meant well rather than a lawyer. In starting up the company, we had made some phone calls to people we knew from our previous employment to see how much interest we could generate in our own enterprise. To our amazement, we had a full route for our pest control company within days.

In an earlier chapter, you'll recall our first battle with the lion—the loss of my dear friend Mark. We were now about to begin our second battle.

May is the busiest month of the year for pest-control work in Northern Michigan, and our first May, in 2006, was a dandy. But just one week into it, I received a phone call, then a visit from a courier carrying legal documents announcing that our former employer would be suing us for more than one million dollars and demanding that we disband and turn over all assets, monies, and equipment to them. Enter, the bear. This battle was waged by a man with an uncontrolled ego, almost unlimited resources, and a level of pride and arrogance seldom seen in Christians … at least real Christians, anyway. The battle would drag on for almost two years, cost him more than $150,000, and cost us more than $60,000 to defend. The only people who made out in this whole deal were the attorneys.

Because the company sued me, Becky, and our corporation, all three of us, at our attorney's recommendation, had to file bankruptcy in the fall of 2007 in an effort to stop the bleeding and make sure the judge didn't throw a million-dollar judgment at us. Just as we were warned, the company sued us in bankruptcy court as well.

There was no reason for either legal action. How could we run an $8 million-a-year company out of business when, in our first year, we were looking at doing only $62,000 in revenue—and only $26,000 of that came from their former customers? Yes, we had agreed when we left the company that we couldn't work for any of their customers for a period of one year following our departure, and if we did, we would face a potential penalty per customer. But this was overkill.

In the end, although they sued us for $1.2 million, we offered $26,000 in cash, and we ended up settling for $12,000 and a four-year ban on every customer they had outside of Leelanau County. It was perfect! Leelanau County was where we did most of that $26,000 that we offered them anyway. Now we were free to serve those customers plus expand as we pleased in the county. Oh, and we saved $14,000 to boot. We got a kick out of that for sure.

If I could go back and redo that whole scenario, I would have waited just two more months to start our company and been free of the one-year agreement. We also both regretted filing for bankruptcy. That threw the previous five years of really hard work on our finances into a tailspin—a bother for another seven years. But the business would prove to be a very rewarding risk, and those seven years would end up being a non-issue overall.

During this time at home, the stress was incredibly hard on Becky, and that broke my heart. She had done absolutely nothing to warrant any of this. But here we were, up to our necks in the pressure of court proceedings, depositions, tons of money going out to pay for legal fees, years of payments to attorneys afterward to try to get things paid off, and the looming potential of being shut down. I would read later on that this kind of stress increases the risk of health issues, including cancer, simply because the immune system is suppressed.

It was amazing to me, though, to watch my wife navigate this season of our lives, move into her role as customer-service rep out of our home while still raising our kids, and growing to become known as the "smile" people sensed over the phone for years to come. How proud I was to have customers in the field say how great it was talking with Becky. She was our customers' first contact and the reason we grew and prospered the way we did those first several years. Of course, once they met me and our sons, our charm put things over the top. At least that's what I told Becky when I got home. She'd smile, kiss me, and grab another phone call.

Pest control for us was a very seasonal affair, and so by late September, things would settle down and the revenue would dry up quickly. To help fill the gap, I was offered a job delivering propane locally during the winters of 2007, 2008, and 2009. I loved that job and worked for a fantastic manager and fellow drivers. I loved driving, I loved seeing results in my work immediately, and because of my abilities behind the wheel, my work ethic, and my self-starting qualities instilled in me by my dad, my boss nicknamed me his "go-to guy."

I would be the one he would call to bail him out of a jam—on a weekend, or late at night, or on overtime any given day. I enjoyed that name and prided myself on making Kevin's job and his day easier. And in turn, he went out of his way to make my job as fun, rewarding, and accommodating as he possibly could. I would work for him again in a heartbeat if the need arose. His secretary, Mickie, was also an awesome lady with a great laugh and sense of humor that Becky and I adored.

My first winter delivering propane followed closely what was supposed to be a two- to three-week gig driving a lifelong friend's big truck over the road while he mended from surgery due to Crone's disease. His family needed the truck to keep moving to help bring in money, and it paid me pretty well, too. Because of a major complication, Ward was back in the hospital—in intensive care—for more than a week hanging on by a thread with full-blown sepsis; he needed another several months to recover. So, I drove his truck to the East Coast and back from June to just before Thanksgiving in 2007.

I was glad to help him out, and it also allowed me to get to know Barry, another truck driver. Ward drove for Barry's company. Barry and I became very good friends, work partners, and fellow business owners, and Becky eventually looked to him as a brother. To this day, Barry is one of my closest friends and one of the greatest human beings I have known. (He is the one who would stand by my side at Becky's memorial.)

So, we had beaten the Lion and just met and overcame the Bear. But we were still unaware of the Goliath that was headed our way.

15]   SOMBER CONVERSATIONS

The year 2009 began as most other years had in our marriage. Our business was growing, and that allowed us to do more dreaming every season. Tim and Andy were out of school and out of the house, one living locally and the other in college. Our Golden died the prior spring, and so we were a one-dog family at the moment, and I was delivering propane. Becky was working on spring letters and enjoying the remodel we had completed last fall on our main level, complete with a new floor, bathroom, and built-in entertainment system. I was due to have my annual physical in January, something I never looked forward to, and Becky was doing her part by making sure I didn't miss it. I would end up owing my life to her and my doctor in just a few short weeks.

During my physical, I asked the doc if he could remove some skin tabs on my underarms and a mole on my chest that had been bothering me. He agreed and began cutting away. The mole had been itching for months and had a skin-colored growth protruding slightly from it. No big deal, I thought. This mole had been around for as long as I could remember, but I had just grown tired of the itching. So off it came, and to my doctor's credit and without me knowing then, he sent if off to the lab for testing. They sent it to a major hospital—one of the nation's leading authorities on melanoma—and my worst fears were realized.

Before I would hear from my doctor, though, Becky's dad would hear from his. He had been having some issues with his bowels, and following a colonoscopy, it was discovered that he had colorectal cancer. This was early February, 2009. He called Becky to tell her that surgery and radiation were scheduled. He would also eventually go through chemo that would just about kill him … and on other days, make him wish he was dead. This was incredibly hard on her dad and hard on Becky. He was three hours away, and there wasn't much that she or I could do to help.

On Valentine's Day, I was delivering propane north of Elk Rapids when my cell phone rang. It was my doctor, and the news wasn't good. He told me that after sending the mole for testing, it was confirmed that I had melanoma. On the K scale—the scale used at that time to determine the depth of the cancer into the dermal tissue, with 5 being the deepest and 1 the best—mine was a 2.5. I was scheduled for surgery in March, during which I would have the remaining mole completely removed, including surrounding tissue to get clean margins. I would also have a sentinel node biopsy to determine if the cancer had spread beyond the site of the mole. I had about three weeks to research my situation, and basically, with a 2.5 tumor, I had a fifty-fifty shot of surviving six months, based on national averages.

Conversations around our dinner table began to get deep and ominous. I had been doing lots of research, so I began preparing Becky and the kids for my possible departure. I'd always been someone who spoke the brutal truth, no matter the situation or the people involved, and this would be no different. I don't like surprises, and I wasn't going to let this surprise any of us. On a day after I shared the news, I remember being in the office when our son Andy came in. He was pretty shaken up. I could tell he had been wrestling with our conversations and needed to vent. It wasn't long before he burst into tears, and we ended up sitting and hugging each other for a very long time. I assured him everything was going to be fine no matter which way this went. It was a conversation we would repeat almost word for word in just a few short weeks.

I began documenting passwords, websites for banking stuff, business decisions that Becky would have to take over, and business decisions that Tim would have to take over. I began encouraging our sons to think about life after dad and how to go on and be my representative each and every day. I also started helping Becky embrace the possibility of needing to open her heart to another to help her with the business, the few sons still at home, and her future life. Those were tough, nearly impossible conversations. Thankfully, I only had a few weeks to ponder all of this before I would know the results of the lymph-node test. This disease has very few survivors once in the lymph nodes—about a five to ten percent survival rate, according to the American Cancer Society's website, which I spent way too much time viewing. It also spreads very quickly and very brutally once beyond the nodes. The main treatment at the time was what doctors described as the most difficult chemo regimen available. I would have to decide whether to give the drugs a shot or just get my affairs in order and get the rest over as fast as possible.

The day of surgery arrived, and Becky was a trooper. She accompanied me into the prep room and was like a rock for me. I know her heart was being crushed, but she never let it show ... not there, anyway. She loved on me, held my hand, hugged me, prayed for me, and reassured me that everything was going to be just fine.

After a couple of hours in surgery and another bit of time in recovery, I woke up and saw Becky walking alongside my bed as they wheeled me down the hallway. I remember hearing her say that the doctor said everything looked good, and although he wouldn't say for sure, he thought the nodes looked clean and the margins clear. Those were some great words to hear. At least

I still had some hope, for a few more days anyway, until they got the lab results from the node biopsies.

So, in just a few more days we would be faced with one of three options—I would be leaving this planet, or I would be fighting the cancer with chemo, or I'd be cancer-free but befriending a good dermatologist for the rest of my life. Of course, since I'm writing this now, it's obvious the nodes were clean and I was free of cancer. I would have to get to the five-year mark, though, before anyone would give me a complete thumbs up. But that came and went as well, and life went on. The love of my life wasn't so fortunate.

16] GOLIATH

Our first battle—losing a dear friend—forced us to trust God for the secret things that passed understanding and to learn the truth of grace and mercy. The second battle included the same but added another element: Let God fight the battles that we didn't start, don't deserve, and have little way of winning on our own.

The final battle would include all of these elements but would add another necessary lesson ... the greatest lesson: The need to forgive God and forgive ourselves, and to believe in His goodness even when the battle seemed lost.

Bud was getting through his ordeal slowly but surely, and I had healed and was ready to jump into pest control for the spring. Becky had turned forty the previous September, and so per her doctor's recommendation, she scheduled her first mammogram in April, just one month after I was cleared of melanoma. During her office visit before her mammogram, her doctor was doing a routine examination of Becky's breasts and thought she felt a lump on the left side.

We had learned earlier that a large number of women have fibrous breasts—breasts with non-cancerous lumps that come and go with monthly cycles and hormonal changes. Becky was one of these women, and so for years, we had noticed such occurrences in each breast. But we had become complacent. We tended to ignore them, assuming they were just the normal monthly thing, and we went on like nothing was wrong.

Becky had the mammogram and a few days later we were called into her doctor's office for a follow up and the test results. Her doctor was about in tears, so we knew the news wasn't good. They had found one lump and it was cancerous. An MRI was scheduled to determine the course of treatment regarding surgery, and that test discovered another lump. It was decided to do a full mastectomy on the left side and leave the right breast untouched because it was clear. During surgery, they would do a sentinel node biopsy on Becky just like they did on me, and they would also get clean margins around the breast. During the exam of the tissue they had removed, they discovered three more tumors undetected by the mammogram and the MRI. That news rocked my world. So many tests, so much technology, and yet, somehow, three out of five tumors were undetected until surgery.

Those first several months of treatment were a frustrating blur. There was the initial surgery, a partial reconstruction of the left breast that would have to be delayed indefinitely because Becky developed scar tissue, the news that the cancer had been found in the lymph nodes, a couple of visits to our first oncologist who had a very uncomfortable and irritating bedside manner, and finally a phone call from his assistant giving us a Stage 4 diagnosis over the phone. Yep, over the phone. And she gave it to me, not Becky. When I asked to speak with the oncologist, I was told that he didn't take phone calls and that I could ask her my question and she would get with him and then back to me. So instead of a question, I gave her a message to pass on. I told her to let him know another office would be calling to have Becky's records transferred over, and we wouldn't be back to their office ever again. She was a bit dumbfounded but obliged.

We never did hear from that first doctor—no phone call, no

letter, nothing. It was disappointing, to say the least. We switched to another local doctor whose specialty was breast cancer. We met with him and learned that we didn't need to start chemo as the first doctor said, because the bone scan confirmed the cancer was in the hip and femur; chemo wouldn't touch it.

Her cancer was hormone-based, and so the first five years the focus was on eliminating estrogen in her body and strengthening the bones the best we could. We had found a competent doctor, devised a plan of attack, and got through the initial surgeries. She would get a port put in that wouldn't get used for almost six years, get a hysterectomy to reduce the amount of medication needed to eliminate estrogen, have four PET scans a year to monitor organ and soft tissue involvement, and get numerous shots, medications, and infusions for bone strength, hormone treatments, and lab work. The medical whirlwind had started, and we were deep into it.

As to Becky's prognosis … we were given the standard survival rate of 24 to 36 months. But Becky never talked about that, and neither did I. From day one, Becky's focus was on everything "but" cancer. That courageous woman was determined that if cancer was going to take her, it was going to be on her and God's terms, and nobody else's. (Becky wasn't the first woman in our family to be diagnosed with breast cancer, by the way. My mom had a mastectomy and most of her lymph nodes in her left arm removed in 1986. She has been cancer-free for 32 years.)

My melanoma, and now Becky's cancer, were not the first times that we'd faced dire challenges with family health issues. James, number five of our six sons, was born in 1994 but was three weeks premature. Once born, it was determined that he had underdeveloped lungs. While under the oxygen hood that first night, he coded. The monitor alarms startled him, and his heart started back up. We learned that he had an underdeveloped flap in the bottom of the esophagus that allowed stomach acid to flow back up the wrong direction, causing some sort of apnea and stopping the heart and breathing. If God hadn't allowed the lung issue, which was potentially fatal, we might have taken him home that first night, and he might have died while we slept.

The lesson learned was that we should never second-guess a circumstance in our life or assume we know the whole story. We should allow God to do His thing in our lives, and trust that He sees the bigger picture and has our best interest in mind. It's called faith, and sometimes it doesn't make sense, and sometimes we just need to close our eyes and hang on.

Just months after seeing our world shatter and our long-term hopes and dreams start to vanish, we encountered a blessing involving our business. I took a look at my heavy-duty truck that was sitting in the driveway, rarely used in winter, and decided we could put a snow plow on it. We surveyed our customers and, sure enough, they said they'd welcome this new snow-clearing service. So almost instantly, our little seasonal company was transformed into a year-round enterprise.

That turned out to be a great financial decision. Just as important, it allowed me amazing flexibility, especially after Tim came on board fulltime. Becky and I were able to go on day dates during a work week whenever the opportunities allowed, stay in and hide on days when things were tough and unrelenting, disappear out of town for a short break here and there, and so much more. We could spend unforgettable and priceless amounts of time together as she fought her illness.

It was literally the vehicle that allowed us to be joined at the hip for however much time we had left, and the finances to enjoy that time and knock some things off the bucket list. God was amazing, my wife a phenome, and our marriage full of exactly what was needed to navigate these new and troubled waters.

By this time, I had started a Caring Bridge blog to share Becky's cancer fight with friends and family and even strangers. The goal was to inform, encourage, and help readers ... but also to allow me a place to express my own thoughts about what was happening.

Here's an entry I posted at about this time:

Speaking of my honey. As many of you know, we had a PET scan last week and a follow up with the oncologist today. But before I go any further, I need to explain the "we" in many of my statements. When I say we have cancer and we had a test and we go to the doctor, I mean it quite literally. The actual cancer may be in Becky's body, but we have it and we are dealing with it. When we were married almost 23 years ago now, we made a commitment to each other in the form of Vows. We committed to be there for each other and with each other through absolutely everything. When we were married our individual lives became one seamless life. We don't have separate bank accounts, separate beds, separate rooms, separate hobbies, separate friends or anything else. We are one flesh and each of our days is all about the unity and the one, not about the individual. That is one of the reasons for a 23-year marriage that has gotten better and better and one of the reasons neither of us has ever been tempted to go outside of it for any type of fulfillment or satisfaction. We made a commitment and we go about everyday fulfilling that commitment.

17]   TRAVEL, SONS, AND MORE

Becky would be the first one to tell you that the first few years of cancer were relatively easy. Emotionally, not always easy. But physically, not bad. We didn't do much other than beat back her estrogen levels and monitor everything else. To Becky's credit, she always was an optimist, always smiling, and she took those first surgeries, tests, scars, discomforts, and unknowns, and focused on living while beating her cancer back to where it came from—hell. As time went on, and the battle worsened, her resolve didn't change, nor did her attitude or smile. But the idea of beating it back to the point of being cancer-free became less of a focal point. Instead, beating it back so she could live another year, month, week, or even day became the more realistic focus.

It was during these first few years that we took as many opportunities as possible to just sit around at parties, or on the front porch of the Walnut Drive home, or at basketball games, and enjoy the company and conversation that went along with hanging out with six amazing sons.

The year 2010 was awesome because we got to be a part of one of Suttons Bay's best basketball seasons ever; two of our sons were on the team. They lost only the first and last game of that season, and the last game was at the Breslin Center at Michigan State University—at the state championship game. What an epic year, and oh what fun Becky had designing signage, baking cookies for the team, and making homemade shirts for everyone that wanted one.

That year was special, too, because we took an amazing vacation out west. It was in the summer. We traveled in two cars hauling eight people and two weeks' worth of supplies. Talk about logistics and efficient planning! We rented a vacation home on the west side of the Grand Teton Mountains at the base of the Grand Targhee Ski Resort for a full week, and truly had the adventure of a lifetime. We hiked, climbed, rode the ski lift to the top of the resort hill, and had a close-up view of the Tetons from the backside. We visited Yellowstone and saw incredible wildlife, and we experienced white-water rafting as a family with the entire raft to ourselves. We had never done anything even remotely like this before.

I have to tell a quick story about the resort. Our vacation home was at an elevation of about 5,000 feet. The top of the resort just a few miles away was at about 7,400 feet. The peak hill was at 10,000 feet. When we got to the resort, I bought round-trip packages, up the chairlifts to the top and back, for $15 a person. To my surprise, everyone got really excited about that, so off we went.

My first job as a sixteen-year-old was working at Sugar Loaf Ski Resort in Leelanau County just eight minutes from my home growing up. One of the perks was free skiing, which I did from time to time. So, I knew my way around a ski resort. However, somehow because of the amazing distraction caused by the view of the Grand Teton mountain range, I didn't notice that when they put us four-wide in the seats, they hadn't lowered the safety bar in front of us. The chairs were eighty feet off the ground because of the sixty feet of snow they get most winters. It was a white-knuckle ride up! My son Stephen eventually realized the problem, reached up, and pulled down the bar. The rest of the trip was less nerve racking.

We got to the top, ungracefully jumped off, and marveled at the magnificent vistas—a bird's-eye view of the Tetons. It was spectacular. And then, too soon, it was time to get back on the chairs and head down. I hollered at everyone to head that way.

Becky turned around and, to all of our surprise, this mild-mannered and soft-spoken woman, who seldom ever swore, said in the most firm and unequivocal voice she'd ever used: "There's no way in hell I'm getting back on that lift."

While at the bottom earlier, I had noticed that if you wanted to hike down, you could … although it was an average of a three-hour trip to do so. Becky must have noticed that hiking was an option, too, because she turned and walked away, down the trail, without the rest of us. Tim and Stephen headed toward the lift and said they'd meet us at the bottom; everyone else just stood and looked at Becky. I spoke up quickly and told everyone that we came up the mountain as a family, and we would go down as one. Boy, did the whining commence! The boys pointed out that the lift was a perfectly good, working machine, that we didn't have water, that none of us had on the right clothing for walking … On and on they went.

In fact, we had a blast on the hike. And we made it down the mountain in ninety minutes. I was so proud of Becky.

After one of the greatest weeks of our lives as a family, we left the beautiful mountain home and traveled to Glacier National Park and drove the Going-to-the-Sun Road. Again, we were overwhelmed by the beauty.

• • • •

So far, I haven't talked about our sons in detail in this book, and you might wonder why. But here is a good spot to do so, because the hike story reminds me of a key point about our marriage. The fact is, our sons have never been the main "story" of my and

Becky's lives. That story has always been Becky and me. That may sound strange, but let me explain.

When I met Becky, we decided to get married and become one in the eyes of God and the world. It was then our family was born—right there in front of that congregation and upon the phrase, "I now pronounce . . ." In that instant, nothing more than the two of us would ever have been needed to complete a family, define it, or give it purpose. We were enough then, and we would be enough after our kids packed up for college and life, and headed out on their own.

So our kids were never the center of our universe. Our marriage and our lives didn't revolve around them. Instead, their lives revolved around ours, with the understanding that we were simply there for a time to train, educate, love, nurture, discipline, and encourage them so we could send them out the door with the best possible chance of succeeding, loving, and living a great life—perhaps a life better than our own.

Our sons have grown to become incredibly resilient, loving, funny, confident, focused, and respected young men. Some are married, some have children, and some are in the process of all of that. Some are professionals, some are blue collar, some are still in school, and some are exploring. But each of them, without exception, is an individual with all of the tools and means necessary to conquer life as we have and pass the legacy of our marriage, our union, our love, our commitment, our faithfulness, and our passion on to their marriages, and to their children, careers, and personal explorations.

In short, Becky and I succeeded in producing Godly young men who will make this world a better place, who will be better men than I've been, and better parents than we were. They are or will be better husbands than I was, and will honor all of their commitments just as I have.

· · · ·

The trip out west was the first family vacation of this scope in our family's history. And it was truly a blessing, because it was made possible by the many, many folks who attended a fund-raising benefit for Becky earlier that spring at the Suttons Bay Schools.

More than 600 people attended, and the money raised was part of almost twenty-seven thousand dollars given to help with Becky's medical bills and health insurance costs. In addition to the benefit, the *Leelanau Enterprise* published an article on Becky and our family, and more donations poured in. Never had we felt such a closeness and greater appreciation for our community as we did then. Our hearts were bursting with gratitude and humility at the level of care our neighbors had shown us.

Because we had never done a trip like this, we decided it would be appropriate to spend some of the money on a family trip. Even though we were just into our second year of Becky's battle, statistically we were looking at just a few more months or maybe a year before things could turn for the worst. That was our mindset: We always planned for the worst but hoped for the best. So that was the impetus for the trip—a bucket-list trip that would provide memories and stories to help sustain us during the coming fight.

Over the next two years, we would take a couple of other family trips. We went to Tennessee to see the Smoky Mountains. It was great fun but much closer and much easier planning and pulling off. It was a shorter getaway but still provided some peace and relaxation. A trip to Florida at the beginning of 2012 had us deciding between traveling more and moving to a warmer climate. We started in Pensacola with a day of exploring the naval base where the Blue Angels reside, watched a practice show, and camped at Fort Pickens Park on the point overlooking the inlet by the naval base and the Gulf of Mexico. The food at the local restaurants was fantastic, and the kids, Becky, and I all had a blast. We worked our way over for a night with great friends, Scott and Tommye, in Jacksonville Beach. From there, we wound up at an RV park very close to the Kennedy Space Center. What a day that was.

James and Jonny had to get back to school as spring break was winding down, so after sending them home, Becky and I were on our own. Oh darn, what would we do? We played in the outdoor heated pool and hot tub. We enjoyed some fine dining out, then pointed the RV south and headed for Marathon in the Keys. The trip was beautiful, the stay amazing, the weather perfect, and the experience priceless. It was a trip we put on our list to do again ... but never would get the opportunity. And that makes me incredibly sad and angry. From this point on, dozens and dozens of visits to hospitals, doctors, and infusions would steadily, annoyingly interfere with almost every other plan we tried to make. The anger and resentment about this nasty disease would get the best of us at times.

To the amazement of doctors, Becky had made it to the thirty-six-month "terminal" date and well beyond. Every year that she celebrated a birthday, the more we believed we could make it to another one. And Becky's perspective on birthdays had changed; our family would get an earful when they complained of getting older. Becky would look at the complainer and simply say, "You know what it means if you're not having any more birthdays, right?" Soon those complaints stopped. Yep, we believed we could make it to another one.

In May of 2014, I sat down with Becky and put her on the spot. As more and more time had passed, I realized how important it was to make sure we weren't missing any travel opportunities. I needed to know if Becky had anything she wanted to do while she still could. We had talked about traveling more. I really wanted to show her some things I had seen with some of the kids while driving the truck. I had mapped several road trips we could do out West, out East, and right around our own Great Lakes region. If we were to start taking long weekends, a week here and a couple weeks there, I thought we could knock some pretty amazing items off our bucket list and enjoy some priceless adventures together, just her and me.

But I also knew that our family was growing, grandkids were on the way, three weddings had been planned for the following summer, and the house we were in wasn't going to accommodate the future Thanksgivings I knew my sweetheart would want to host. In fact, the last two seasons we had been blessed with the use of a gorgeous home complete with gourmet kitchen and room for dozens on Stony Point, compliments of those great friends in Jacksonville. And as fun and convenient as that was, it wasn't Becky's kitchen, and I knew she had been thinking about that, too.

After some give and take, some hemming and hawing, and lots of her asking "what do *you* think?" I finally made her tell me just what *she* wanted, not what she thought *we* wanted. And, for the first time in my life with her, she gave me a selfish answer: She wanted a bigger house with a large living room, a kitchen for our whole family, a barn for some animals someday, and a covered front porch where she could sit and rock her grandbabies. I think deep down in my soul that was my dream, too. I wanted to travel, sure, but once she spoke those words, in that order, we both teared up and grabbed each other close. I promised her I was going to make this happen while we still could.

It was early May, and our busy season was ramping up, so I had my hands full. I really didn't think much could happen on the new house for a month or more, but I wanted to call my credit union to get some realistic numbers … to see what our possibilities were, if any. To my surprise, he gave us a pretty healthy number and some very doable guidelines, granting us the go-ahead to start shopping.

This is where the story gets really cool. I had talked with the credit union on a Monday. By Wednesday, I had looked on line at all kinds of homes in our area in that price range. I called a realtor I knew, Teddy Lockwood, and asked if he could get us into a couple of those homes just so we could see what our money could buy. Neither of them was ideal and would end up not being of interest to us, but we now had a better idea of the market. After walking through those two homes on Friday morning of that same week, I took Becky for a ride to curbside-shop a couple more listings I had noticed online. One was an instant "no," but the other one had promise. We drove partway up the drive so we didn't disturb the folks who were there, gazed out our windows, and began to talk about all of the house's potential. We called the realtor back and asked if we could see it the following morning, Saturday. He arranged it.

We looked at the home, explored the property a bit, and talked about all the things we could do after the current owner removed his stuff. We followed Ted back to his office, drew up an offer that was $20,000 less than the asking price, signed the paperwork, and headed for an early Mother's Day party at my late grandmother's house with my mom, my sisters, Becky, and our sons.

About two hours later, Ted called and informed us the owner had accepted the offer without a counter and to come back to his office as soon as we could to sign the purchase agreement. Becky and I stood facing each other for a moment and exclaimed, almost in stereo, "What have we done?" It had been only six days since we discussed the idea of a new house and here we were, signing a purchase agreement to buy a house on fifteen acres that was just a mile from where I grew up. How great was that? More fitting a question: How scary was that?

Two days later, Ted came to our current home to take pictures, take care of a sellers' agreement, and get our home listed. He also gave us some pointers on making the house ready to sell. Boy, did we have our work cut out for us. Remember, this was our busy season!

It was Tuesday evening, the house was online, and the next day we had our first showing. Three days later, on Saturday, we had two more showings, and by Sunday afternoon—just one week after we had signed a purchase agreement on our new home— we had a full-price offer on ours with a second offer ready should the first one fall through. Thirty days later, we moved to White Road, into our dream home with a covered front porch that would come to be a place of recovery, dreams, reminiscing, and visits with our favorite people ... a place to make precious memories. Only God could orchestrate such a string of events, and only God knew just how important this home would be.

18] A BATTLE BEGINS

As great as it's been to write about the fun we had purchasing our new home, it's time to deal with the title of this chapter—a battle that started right in the middle of the front porch ... the one place my sweet Becky dreamed of having in her house our entire marriage.

One thing we loved to do in our new home was spend time in the hot tub out back and then come inside, rinse off, put pajamas on, and go sit on the porch in the dark and listen to the night creatures. We would cuddle, smooch, maybe get a little frisky from time to time, but mostly we just sat there and soaked in life together. We were living our dream, and we couldn't be happier.

On this night, October 3, 2014, it was unseasonably warm, almost 70. It was about 11 p.m. and earlier that day I had stacked some split firewood on the outside edge of the porch to carry inside the next day. I never gave it a second thought. I was already out on the porch in my chair, anxiously waiting for Becky to join me so we could watch a lightning storm roll in and soak up the warm air that was forecast to vacate the region in just a few hours.

As she stepped out the door, swung it closed, and turned to head my way, she caught her right toe on the end of that stack of wood and tripped, landing on the floor of the porch in a heap. I ran over to help, but as soon as I touched her, I could tell she was in deep pain; there would be no attempts from me to move her. I ran inside, grabbed my phone, and dialed 911. Becky was sure she had broken something, and she did—her femur, just below the hip. It was the worst pain she'd ever felt, which was saying something considering how much she'd been through already.

I learned in the weeks that followed that many people actually die from the trauma of a broken femur. Becky told our son Stephen on one occasion that she felt like all the years of bone pain resulting from her spreading cancer and the side effects of the medicines had prepared her to withstand the brutality of the pain she experienced lying on the front porch of her dreams. That broke Stephen's heart to know his mom was hurting that much.

Not a minute after I hung up the phone, I was surprised when two county deputies sped into the driveway. They had been cruising down the highway close to our home when the call came in and wasted no time in getting to us. Several hours and lots of help later, we were in recovery at our local hospital. Becky was scheduled to have a rod put in from her knee to her hip.

The fall was a major setback for Becky ... a blow not just to her physically but emotionally as well. From time to time in the few years prior to the injury, Becky had struggled greatly with her self-esteem. It began when she lost a breast and tried to have it reconstructed, only to have to stop partway through the process and leave it as it was. She would also have the other breast tweaked a bit to try and match the new one, but having not been able to finish that one, too, left both "out of sync," so to speak.

Becky was also having trouble keeping weight off during those first few years—a result of hormone imbalances, medications, reduced mobility, and a general lack of energy. It all accumulated into a major blow to her self-worth. I was doing my best to reassure her and focus our attention elsewhere. Some days it worked; on others, my effort fell on deaf ears. Becky just didn't feel beautiful anymore, she didn't feel sexual anymore, and she didn't have the desire to even try on days when she did feel good. She had taken a beating emotionally, physically, and mentally and was beginning to question whether it was all worth it.

She knew how badly I still wanted to make love to her and so, on nights or afternoons (if the kids were gone) when she was feeling better than normal, she would do everything she could to enjoy a part of our relationship that had grown distant because of this horrible disease. And each time we would enjoy those moments, she would always say to me, with tears in her eyes, "I wish we could do this more."

It was during these final three to four years that Becky and I would transition from making love with our bodies to making love to each other's hearts and souls. We would learn to sit and speak things to each other that gave life, purpose, sensuality, and longing. We would just sit and hold each other, caressing, rubbing, and massaging areas that hurt or stung or were fatigued. We would talk intimately about our love for each other and how blessed and fortunate we were to still be together and have our family and friends. To have the home we did. To have the medical benefits we did. To have the income we did, and so on. That became the picture of our love-making. Once in a while, she would get a twinkle in her eye and whisper something amazing in my ear and moments later she would be blessing my life in a way that only she had ever done ... and vice versa. Those moments would become farther and fewer between as time went on, but our love would only grow and our commitments to each other only deepen.

All those years ago, we had learned to love deeply and care completely, and that was proving to be priceless as we moved into the final chapters of our love story. It would be that radiance that so many would comment on while they shared in our journey. It would be the reason our love story would have the impact on others that it did. We had learned to love each other just as God loves us. We had learned to love with our whole hearts, deep from within our beings when our bodies and our emotions were getting the better of us.

After spending about three days in the hospital, Becky was recovering fairly well from the broken femur. But, secretly, I felt shattered. Not wanting to burden her with trying to help me with something, I wouldn't tell her this for another two years: I blamed myself—I put the wood there—and still blame myself for the decline in health Becky faced over the next two years. It was that injury that ultimately opened up a pathway for the cancer to invade the bone marrow, for her body to be weakened and vulnerable, for the influenza she would get just three months later, and for each and every transfusion she would get to keep her hemoglobin at necessary levels.

Eventually, I did break down and tried my best to apologize for failing her and causing her broken leg. Her injury, I felt, was squarely on my shoulders. My negligence had caused this avalanche of pain and suffering. My negligence ended any chance of Becky being able to beat this thing, or at least get the years we were hoping to get. Of course, I know it's impossible to know what caused what. But there is simply no escaping the fact that shortly after the accident, Becky's health began going south in a hurry. She never would make a recovery. That's on me, and no one will ever convince me otherwise.

One evening in November, after Becky came home to recover, I was in watching a late-night infomercial while she was in the dining room working on a holiday project. The infomercial happened to be for Cancer Treatment Centers of America. I watched about five minutes of it and asked Becky if she could come in and finish it with me.

We had been getting progressively more frustrated with our local oncologist. Every time we saw him, we were getting rushed through the office faster and faster, like a herd of dairy cows on their way to the stanchions. We felt like we couldn't talk with him, mostly because as we sat in the room waiting, we would usually hear him getting after one of the staff for overbooking or forgetting to tell him about an appointment. The local hospital had purchased his practice a couple months prior, and the new systems, new format, and new ways were frustrating everyone in the office, as well as we patients. It was also becoming very clear that he was in a reactive rather than proactive mode with us. It seemed like he was waiting for something to happen so he could figure out what to do, and that wasn't sitting well with me.

At the end of the infomercial, I asked Becky what she thought and her response was, "Can I call them?" I was thrilled. Becky dialed the number, and fifteen minutes later we had an appointment at Cancer Treatment Centers of America in Zion, Illinois, just a few miles south of the Wisconsin border and right on Lake Michigan.

The descriptions of the forty-plus trips we would make to this hospital for Becky's care over the coming two years could fill another book. But what is most important is that I credit CTCA with getting us almost another two years together. It was also CTCA that never used the word "terminal," "death," or "dying"— not even once, even when that news was given through other, gentler words just twenty-one days before her life would end. This was in sharp contrast to what we had heard at our local hospital. There, from day one in 2009, every doctor, nurse, attendant, ER doc, and radiation technician would seem to go out of their way to remind us that we were dealing with a terminal disease, and that this thing would take her life, eventually.

This new tone would be a defining difference in care and would give us strength as we faced the intense battles ahead.

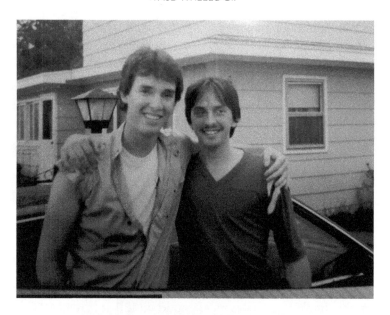

Summer 1985 and my great friend Mark on the right.

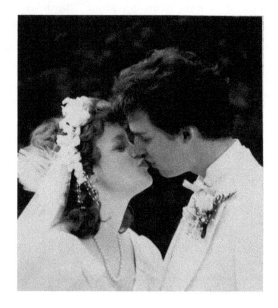

April 11th, 1987. Day 1 of our 30-year marriage.

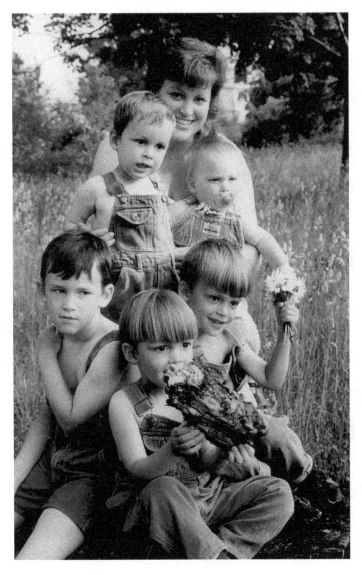

Becky with our first 5 of 6 sons in the summer of 1995.

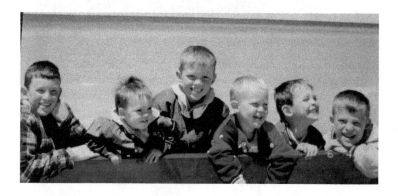

Empire beach, fall of 1998.

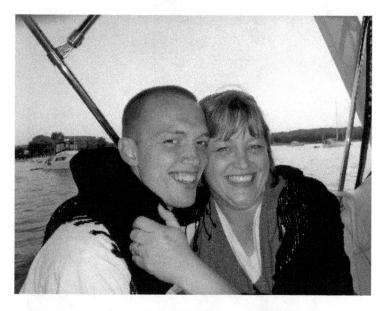

Becky and son number 3, David. Grand Traverse Bay,
Cherry Festival 2011.

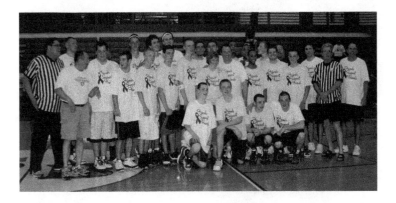

Benefit basketball game for Becky at Suttons Bay High School gymnasium, April 2010.

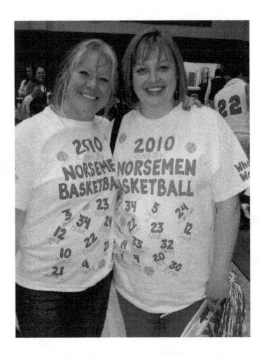

Becky and great friend Karen sporting shirts Becky made for our boys' varsity basketball team on their way to the state championship game in Lansing.

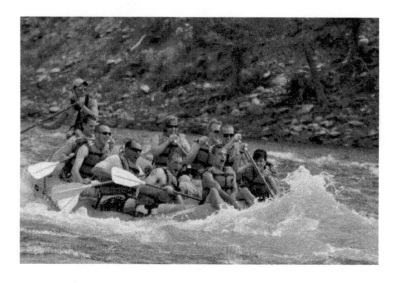

Whitewater rafting in the Yellowstone River 2010.
Whole raft to ourselves.

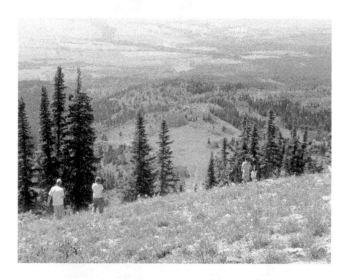

The family hike down the ski hill at Grand Targhee Ski Resort
2010, backside of the Grand Tetons.

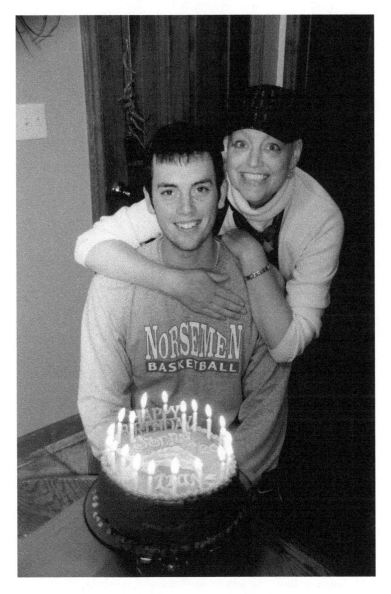

Becky and our youngest, Jonny, on his 20th.

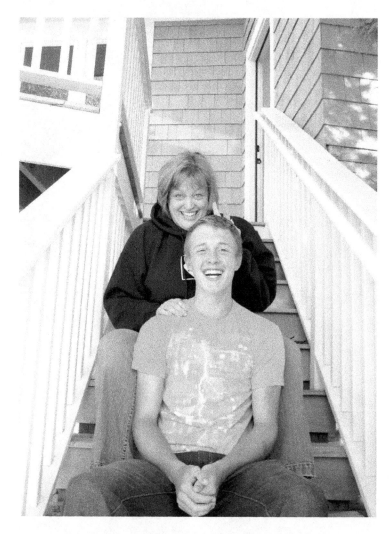

Senior picture time with James, number 5, and Becky, 2013.

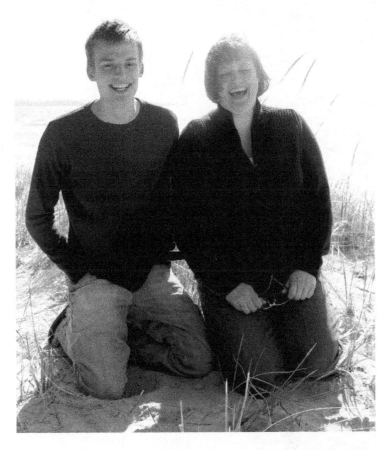

Senior picture time on the shores of Lake Michigan at Glen Haven with Andy, son number 2, 2008.

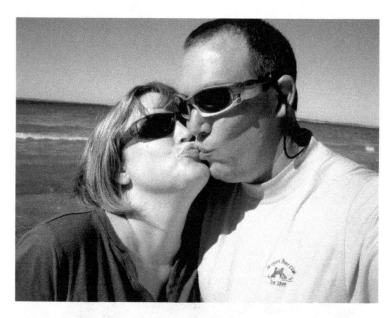

Smooching on the shores of Lake Michigan at Port Oneida 2010.

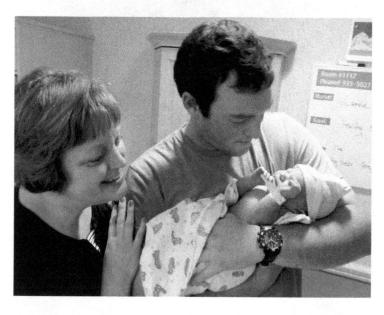

One proud grandma, our oldest Tim, and his first child, Alora, 2014.

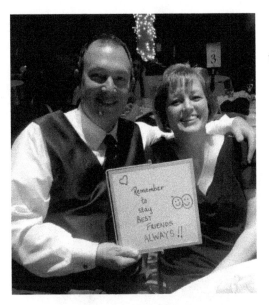

Enjoying a son's wedding reception in 2015, the year we thought we'd lose her.

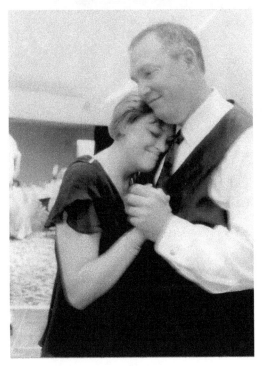

Holding Becky and enjoying our favorite pastime in 2015.

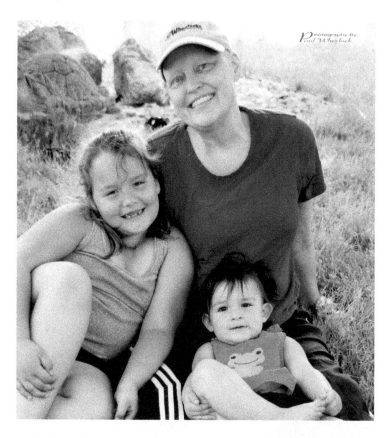

Araya and Alora helping Becky with flowers in the spring of 2016.

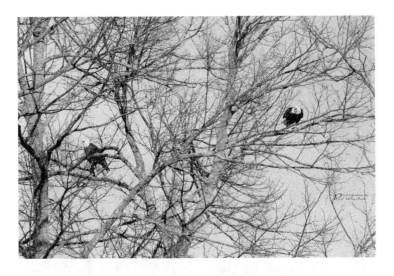

January 1, 2016, just moments after we began planning
our anniversary party from our living room window.

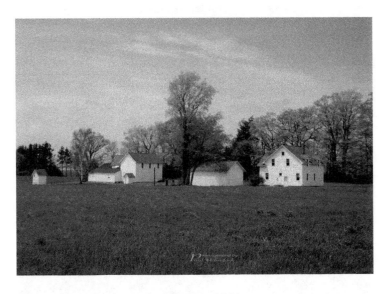

Port Oneida, 2016.

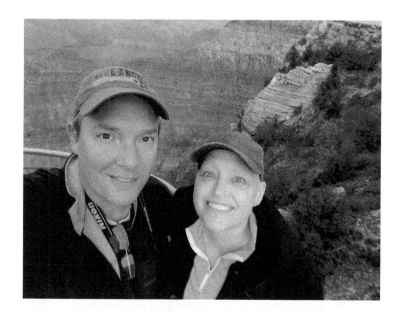

One last bucket list trip, fall of 2016.

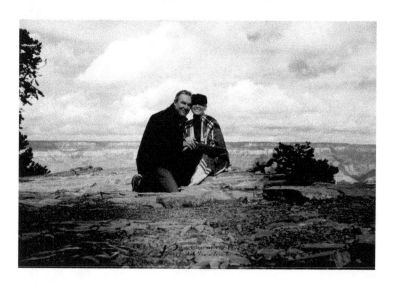

Grand Canyon, fall of 2016.

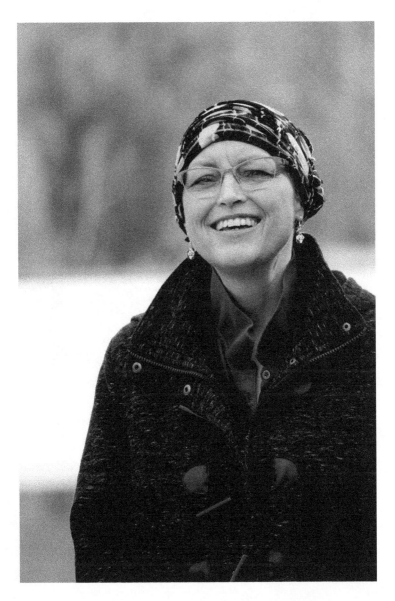

February 2017. The last day that Becky felt good.

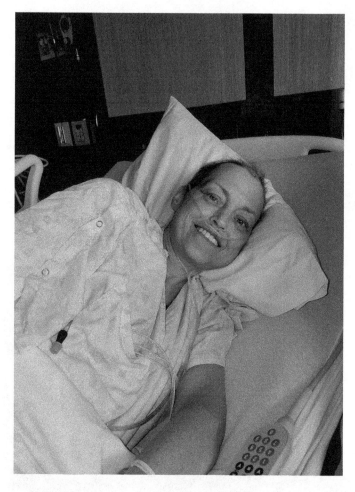

April 4, 2017—the day after we got the devastating news . . .
and still the smile!

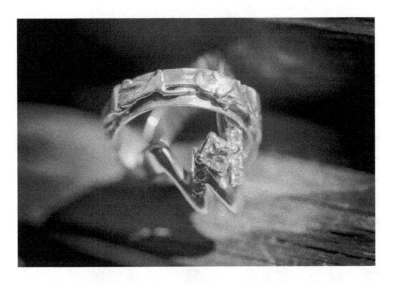

Our rings symbolizing our hearts on our thirtieth-anniversary celebration day, 2017.

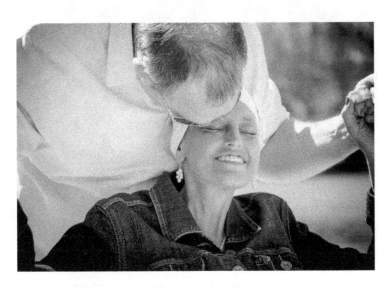

Celebration day, April 2017, at the reception venue.

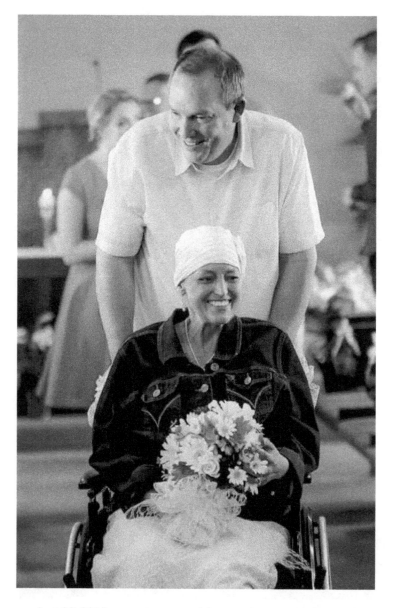

April 22, 2017 . . . anniversary celebration day . . . and the smile!

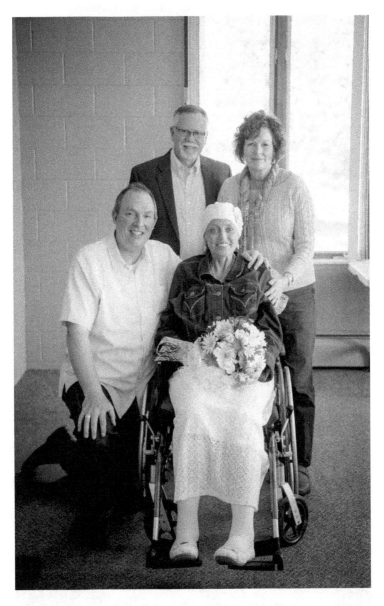

Pastor Keith and Robin Huffman minutes before the ceremony,
April 22, 2017.

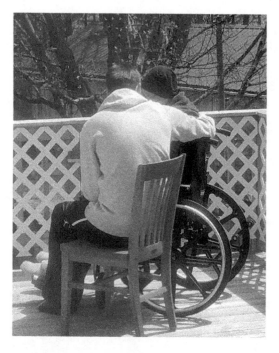

Monday, April 24, 2017. Stephen trying to tell his mom goodbye.

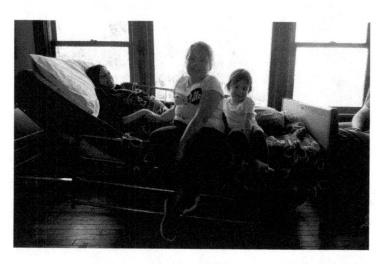

Grandkids' last visit with grandma, April 24, 2017.

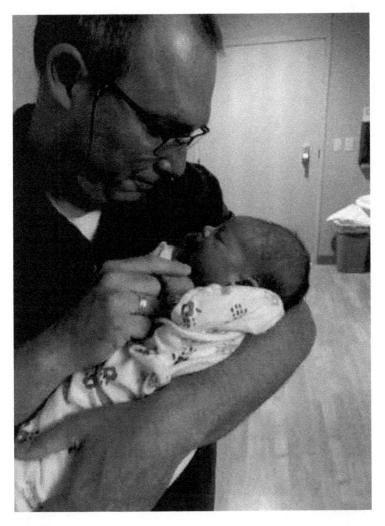

Proud grandpa holding his first grandson, June 1, 2017, as a widower.

19]   WHAT A YEAR!

When we arrived at CTCA the first time, we were greeted with warmth, care, and genuine excitement that we had come all the way from Michigan. Our first day there would prove amazing.

At home, it took weeks and months to get tests done, diagnoses made, and treatment plans put in place. And in order to coordinate everything, we had to travel to offices all over town, seeing multiple people in multiple locations, and—with a few exceptions—felt that we weren't much more than cattle. Oh, how different the story was at CTCA. Within just a few hours, we had met with each department involved with our care. And I say "our" on purpose. The staff at CTCA was focused on treating the patient and the caregiver and providing anything either of us needed. Becky and I were husband and wife. This was *our* cancer, and it was refreshing to be at a place that understood that view.

The meeting with our first doctor—an internist responsible for gathering all of Becky's medical records for the past forty years—was amazing. She had everything. The process was seamless. We simply had to confirm this and that. And the best part? Based on all they had read, viewed, and gone over, they already had a plan of attack and just needed to introduce us to the players—the ones who would do their best to sustain as much life in Becky's body as they could while providing the highest level of comfort. This would prove to be challenging, but the people at CTCA never gave up, never stopped, and never uttered any word of defeat of any kind, even when they privately knew the worst.

Just a couple of months after we began our journey at CTCA, Becky came down with influenza. It was January 2015, and this was the year that our family as well as our loved ones began preparing for what we were sure would be the end. During this year, we traveled to Illinois every couple of weeks. On a couple of occasions, Becky would spend a week in the hospital. When they found that the cancer had spread to her bone marrow, she had to undergo brutal tests. All the while, I watched as her weight began to drop and her body became even more frail and withered.

This was also the year that, because of the bone-marrow issues, Becky had to endure countless blood transfusions in an attempt to keep her alive and fighting. Her body and the cancer were destroying her hemoglobin faster than she could produce it. Those who know about hemoglobin levels are aware that you need to be somewhere between eleven and fourteen, if you're a woman, to be healthy and strong. A transfusion wouldn't be ordered until the levels were eight or under. Most people under eight are bedridden or at least confined to home where they can rest and try to cope with very low energy, both physically and mentally. But not Becky.

We attended our son's wedding in Illinois—a ceremony that was followed by a lengthy brunch—only to find out the next day that Becky's hemoglobin was just over six. Nothing could keep this woman down! Becky had committed to living her life in spite of this raging disease, and that's just what she was doing.

The wedding was in March and came as a surprise to us. Andy had arranged everything for his fiancée, Jessica. You see, they needed to move in together and pool their resources and wanted to combine their efforts going forward. But they also didn't want to ruin what had been a perfect relationship thus far.

Earlier in this story, you'll recall how I preached to our sons about understanding the importance and preciousness of virginity and the gift it is to a future mate. I was very proud to hear Andy tell me that this was the reason for the surprise wedding. Jessica thought they were just exchanging vows and making it legal, but Andy had invited Becky and I along with Jessica's parents and several close friends to attend. Andy had listened to my council all those years, and they were starting things right, and we couldn't have been more proud. They would have a larger, more all-encompassing wedding for the entire family and countless friends in Wisconsin later that summer.

Before they would have that second go-round, though, two of Andy's brothers would also have their turn at saying "I do".

James, son number five, (and yes, we've had to number them over the years to make it easier for folks to relate to what we were telling them), would marry his high school sweetheart, Megan, in mid-July. Just two weeks later, our oldest son, Tim, would marry a wonderful lady with a beautiful and sweet daughter—our first granddaughter—Araya. Tim and Teia would tie the knot in Petoskey and James and Megan in Traverse City. Andy and Jessica would follow them in mid-August in Wisconsin, and just like that, three of our six sons were married.

During what proved to be six amazing and jam-packed weeks, Becky was hanging on by a thread. On top of the transfusions to keep her blood levels stable, she had also begun a grueling chemo regimen that caused her to throw up and barely function from lack of energy. Instead of feeling sorry for herself, though, Becky was simply frustrated that she wasn't able to do more to help with the festivities. Anyone who has known Becky for even five minutes knows how much she enjoyed creating, fixing, preparing, organizing, and being a part of parties, celebrations, and holidays. She lived for stuff like this, and everyone knew it, including her daughters-in-law. And to their credit—and even though they knew how sick and weak she was—they let her help where she could, asked her about ideas, tapped her for advice and wisdom, and made her feel as much a part of things as she could be.

As for me, I had the greatest job of all. I was able to be by Becky's side every day of this entire year. Every day, without exception. I was able to help her when she wasn't able to help herself. I watched her dance with our sons, hoping it wasn't the last time but thinking it might be. I got to dance with her myself and hold her as close as I did that very first time in January 1985. Having been married twenty-eight years, we were able to stay on the dance floor for an extra-long time for the longest marriage dance. And I was so proud we were there. With so many divorces on both sides of our families, and so many unhappy marriages that we witnessed day after day, Becky and I were able to be out there, madly and deeply in love and hanging on to every step, every note of the song, and soaking as much in as we could … both of us scared to death it may be our last dance but thankful to the core that we were there.

20]   GOD'S AMAZING GRACE

One of my favorite nuggets from church so many years ago was the definition of grace and mercy that was shared by various ministers from the pulpit. *Grace affords us the things we absolutely do not deserve, and mercy spares us from those that we do.* And thank God for both. It's grace that God affords us when we fall short—when we fail and when we sin, no matter what the sin or to whom we sin— and its grace that God has also commanded us to give to others in the form of forgiveness, love, patience, and kindness.

I remember this when I think of our families—those who have enriched our lives and been an absolute rock for Becky and me during our cancer battle. In fact, our lives would have suffered and been much worse had it not been for all the help, support, encouragement, prayers, time spent, and resources offered by those closest to us.

Becky's dad, Bud, made it a point to call her several times a week ever since her diagnosis. And I can't tell you how much that impacted her life, especially during those final years. His wife, Emily, loves to hand-write notes and once in a while would send one down from the U.P. It would make Becky's day.

For his part, Bud was always ready to help in any way he could and was always bringing goodies down from the U.P. when he and Emily visited. There was the hand-built rocking horse and cradle he made for us in 1989, the trailer for the lawn tractor that he got us for a house-warming gift, the homemade pies from the neighbors, and even a blueberry pie from a bakery in Paradise that they picked up passing through on their way to Suttons Bay. Bud and Emily were always thinking of us, doing any and all they could, and—most important—never giving up on Becky during all her years of fighting.

I remember a very critical and important moment in our marriage with regard to Becky's dad. I don't remember exactly what year it was, but I remember the details. Becky was talking with her dad on the phone as she had many times before, and at the end of every conversation she would always tell him, "I love you." But on this particular phone call, Bud ended the call by uttering those same words back to her. I remember Becky hanging up the phone, turning to me, and beginning to cry. I could tell they were tears of joy, but I didn't have a clue as to why.

She told me that this was the first time she had heard her dad say those words. In thirty some years, she had never heard him say it to her, her brother, or her mother. While she never doubted that he loved her, to hear him say it for the first time nearly brought her to her knees in thanksgiving to God. That was a defining moment in her relationship with her dad and one that would help both of them become more open in their communication, something that became more and more necessary as time went on.

There was a time right after my folks were divorced that I had difficulty with any kind of relationship with my mom. I didn't like her, didn't want to see her, and surely didn't want to talk to her. I'm sure she knew that and knew why. It would take a few years before we started talking again, and as time went on, God's grace began to pour over both of us. Before too long, we were talking, laughing, visiting, and getting on with our lives in spite of all the hurt and disappointment. And what a blessing that was to her mom, my grandma. We were able to mend a semi-broken family and enjoy the remaining years that grandma had on this earth and celebrate her life together.

After my grandmother passed away, just a month before we moved into our dream home, Becky and I thought for sure my mom would head south to my youngest sister Wendi's area of the state. No one would have been surprised; in fact, we were assuming it would happen. What surprised us was the lack of a "For Sale" sign in the front yard and any talk about a move. It was a couple of years after grandma passed before I asked mom why she was still here. Her response made me and Becky cry. My mom told me that as long as Becky and I weren't traveling and would be staying closer to home, she was determined to stay and not miss any opportunity to be with us.

Boy, did I feel terrible after I thought about this for a time. All these years with my mom only living ten minutes away and I never had a clue as to why she was sticking around and—worse—never made much of an effort to include her in more of what we did. I'm glad to report that as the years went on and over those final months and weeks, my mom was a huge part of our lives and helped in ways that only a mother can.

No matter how old a girl gets, how many kids she has, or how great the marriage to her husband is, a girl always loves having her mother around. For reasons I won't go into (or understand most of the time), Becky didn't have that with her biological mom. Her mom loved her, no doubt, but their relationship was often, if not mostly, backward. And as time continued, Becky instead found herself leaning on my mom for the stuff that only a mother can give: unconditional love and support, emotional encouragement, and a soft voice of affirmation and comfort. My mom—the only person who shed more tears than me when Becky passed—filled that gap and became an incredibly precious gift to Becky. They needed each other in ways that only a daughter and mother can need, and for that we were both eternally grateful.

When Becky and I bought our dream home in 2014, we moved in just one mile from where I was living the day we met—the same place my dad still lives with his new wife Jean of almost twenty years. My dad was far from perfect as I was growing up. I'm sure he would be the first to admit it. But one thing I realized several years back and would share often with Becky was how glad I was that we were becoming close in our older years instead of being close early on and then drifting apart.

I've always had the utmost respect for my dad and have told countless people over the years that I've never met anyone with more integrity, honesty, or loyalty. He may have been a bit lacking in the nurturing and loving department for a lot of years, but he had the other good stuff locked down.

One thing my dad and I never had an issue with was trust. No matter the state of our relationship over the years, we've always been able to trust each other. And the older I've gotten—and with each son Becky and I had—the value of trust and its unbreakable bond would grow and become more precious. I still shake my head sometimes when I think about things that irk me, but the older I get—and after spending the last nine years focusing on just the very best life has to offer—I don't have the energy to go down many of the roads that used to irritate and bewilder me. I've decided to leave that stuff for God and let Him deal with it. Today, my dad and I are pretty tight. And what a rock he's been in this journey, both he and his wife. Countless hours of help, support, errand-running, phone calls, encouraging words, front-porch sits just to chat and enjoy each other's company, and so much more.

I could go on, but the point I'm trying to convey is that without grace, none of us are worthy of a single smile, pat on the back, or encouraging word. And when we realize just how amazing grace really is and extend it to those around us—especially those who have hurt us—we end up receiving it back, tenfold. We really can't lose when we extend a hand of kindness, mercy, and forgiveness. When we do that, we open ourselves up to receive that from God and place ourselves directly in the path of His provisions and love—plus we all sleep better at night when we've done the right and loving thing.

I would be remiss if I also didn't take a moment to mention some of the local doctors and people in the hospital. Even though our experience with our local hospital and the surrounding cancer services had been less than stellar, we still encountered some amazing individuals during this part of the journey.

The nursing staff, for instance, was the silver lining in the dark cloud. The infusion team … the amazing lab ladies at Thirlby Clinic who Becky grew so close to over the years … the pharmacists who became friends and encouragers day after day and week after week … the outstanding care we received with Dr. Thomas and the plastic surgery team early on … and the wonderful nursing staff at what was once Traverse Hematology and Oncology. These ladies made us feel important and cared for even when the rest of the process made us feel like just another cancer case.

One of the many and repeating conversations Becky and I had over the nine years centered on what I would do after Becky was gone. She tried so many times to get me to promise to go on living my life to the fullest. She specifically begged me to promise her that I would find another amazing woman and allow God to build another story of incredible love and life. But no matter how hard she tried to get me to make that promise, all I could do was smile and let her know I'd be okay. I couldn't go that extra bit and promise her I'd love another … not while she was alive and looking into my eyes, anyway. Still, Becky didn't stop pouring grace on me. She gave me permission to move on, love, and live again.

And then there was the grace found in the house, the business, the healthy sons, the healthy grandkids, the amazing daughters-in-law, the loyal and caring customers, and the outstanding medical team at CTCA.

On and on I could go. But the point is this: Our lives, this exhilarating journey that God allowed Becky and me to travel together, have been soaked in grace from the start. Through God's grace, I've been blessed with a woman I did not deserve and allowed the privilege to live a life full of love, goodness, richness—and her—each and every day. And for that I am eternally thankful and overwhelmingly humbled.

21]   THE BATTLE'S END IN SIGHT

After an unbelievably challenging and debilitating year, we approached 2016 a bit differently. Neither of us noticed it at first and didn't spend a lot of time talking about it, but we found ourselves talking less about the future and more about short-term things—upcoming holidays, anniversaries, the next round of treatment or tests, and Becky's week-to-week lab numbers. Without noticing at first, our life had transformed to a day-to-day existence. Becky would spend more time talking about near-term things and little fun projects with the kids instead of future trips and bucket-list items.

Looking back on it now, and whether she was doing it purposely or not, Becky seemed to be preparing for the battle to get tougher. The fatigue and suffering she had endured for the past eight years was beginning to take its toll on her physically and emotionally. Judging by all the hospital bills, medical records, journal entries, and almost two years of texts between her and I—all things that I've saved—the preceding couple of years were the worst. It's still hard to comprehend, without crying and feeling like I failed her, how much of her life was consumed with medical issues.

For two complete years, there was lab work every week and seven- to nine-hour drives to CTCA at least once every month.

Becky broke her leg and was down for weeks, recovering. There were two bouts of influenza, a hysterectomy, an infected port that put her in the hospital for a week, fighting to survive. Hair loss and then hair growth, only to watch it fall out again. Bone pain everywhere and all the time. Swelling in her lower extremities, monthly urinary tract infections, bi-weekly infusions, chemotherapy, and enough pain medicine to put an elephant to sleep.

By early 2016, what Becky had endured over the past eight years was beginning to show in her level of fatigue, the number of naps she would take, the amount of time she could be on her feet, and the depth and length of conversations she would be able to have with those closest to her. The disease was slowly but surely taking over, and we were unwittingly beginning to prepare for the final push.

One of the conversations Becky and I frequently centered on was the notion of praying for healing. We were both God-fearing, Jesus-loving and Bible-believing Christians who knew what the scriptures said about healing. We also knew how we both felt … and we were on the same page.

Neither of us, since the first diagnosis, had ever stopped and asked God to heal her. Some of my church friends are probably reading this right now and gasping, thinking "Well, no wonder she died." And those people would be completely and utterly wrong.

One way that God taught Becky and me about who He is and what He desires from us was to use our positions as parents as a model. The Bible tells us that God is the same yesterday, today, and forever. He created us in His image and His likeness, and He said *as it is in Heaven, so it is on Earth*. The scriptures showed us that God viewed His relationship with us much like He wanted us to view our relationship with our own children.

Never in twenty-eight years as parents did Becky or I ever ask, demand, or even suggest that our children walk in the door, drop to their knees, and begin praying to us to meet their needs, to provide a job, money, or to bring them food, provide them shelter or medicine. We never did. We didn't have to. As parents, your provisions and the protection of your children are an unquestionable and assumed part of the package. Our children had faith that we would do what needed to be done for them. They didn't have to pray for it. They just knew it inherently, before even knowing the meaning of the word.

That is exactly how Becky and I approached her diagnosis. No one had to convince us that God could heal Becky of this disease. We knew He could, without exception. No one had to convince us that God would provide the strength, the peace, and the grace to walk this journey together, no matter the outcome. We just knew He would. In our hearts and deep within our souls, we knew and accepted that He would do what was best and that life would go on, either here on Earth or in paradise. After all, even Jesus had that moment. Remember on the cross when he cried out to God and wondered why He had forsaken Him? And remember when Jesus spoke to the thief next to him during the crucifixion and said to him, "I tell you the truth, today you will be with me in paradise." Do you believe that Jesus believed and knew God could heal Him? Of course.

What did Jesus pray instead in the Garden of Gethsemane?

"Please Father, if there is any way to take this cup from me, but never the less, not my will but your will be done."

Becky and I knew full well God could heal her at any minute from head to toe. As a matter of fact, he had already done it two other times in her life:

The first was when Becky was in her mother's womb and it was determined that she would be an RH baby—a natal disease—and that she would be born severely retarded. Her parents were told they should plan on giving Becky up for institutional care as soon as she was born, because she would never be able to care for herself or be anything more than a child, mentally, her entire life. Thankfully, her parents declined and took her home. I think it's safe to say that God handled that one pretty well.

The second time involved a staph infection in Becky's back when she was a teenager. It put her in the hospital for a month and almost killed her. After exploratory surgeries, tons of medicines, and probe after probe, no one could find any cause for the infection or give any plausible explanation for why it had suddenly gone away. Again, God could and did heal her.

But why those two times and not now? Great questions ... questions that will have to wait to be answered when we are face to face with Him and can comprehend what He is saying. Becky and I resolved in our hearts that we would allow God to do what He was going to do in and through each of us during this battle. We would accept whatever outcome He determined. We knew and believed He could see the beginning from the end, and we knew He was less concerned about us than using us to help others find their way to Him.

In other words, our tickets were already purchased and punched when we said yes to Jesus. Our destiny was set, and there would be nothing to fear in death and dying. It was our job—our privilege and desire—to go about living, doing, and being what God needed us to be to each other, our families and our community.

If you could read the hundreds of cards I received in the weeks following Becky's death, hear about the tens of thousands of people who read her obituary, or speak with the hundreds that came to her memorial, you would quickly see that her impact was so much bigger than we ever dreamed. By going through this horrible process, she would provide an uplifting and everlasting story to people we would never even meet. And that, folks, is called the big picture and why we must be willing to just go with it and trust that God is putting the puzzle together perfectly, and the finished product will be a masterpiece of epic proportions and eternal value.

22]   LET'S PLAN A PARTY

A while back we had inherited a couple of swivel rockers that we placed in front of our living room window. The view overlooked the north valley, apple trees, bird feeders, and a few massive trees. It also allowed us a fantastic and comfortable vantage point to watch a pair of eagles on January 1, 2016.

Becky and I loved sitting in those chairs, facing each other while we drank coffee and dreamed. She would always have a notebook or notepad close by and was always jotting down ideas, recipes, poems, scripture verses, cute little sayings, shopping lists, and anything else you could imagine. She loved to write, and I'm glad she did ... especially now.

The past few weeks without her have been made a bit easier as I'm finding notes in every corner of the house, in every cupboard, drawer, and every shelf. I can actually hear her voice when reading them, like she's speaking to me while I read. I love her handwriting, always have. All of these notebooks and notepads full of stuff is a treasure hunt. Even an old grocery list is suddenly an irreplaceable nugget of gold. I look forward to rainy days so I can stay inside and go through her writings looking for that next nugget without feeling guilty about not being outside enjoying the summer weather. (We make the most of those nice days in Northern Michigan, because winters tend to be long, dark. Rainy summer days are when we get inside chores done: go shopping, get groceries, and catch up on family visits.)

Sitting in those window rockers one early-April morning, Becky and I were talking about our upcoming anniversary, April 11, marking twenty-nine years.

Becky's eyes lit up as she grabbed for her trusty notebook—the big one, so I knew a lot of ideas were coming. She looked at me with her usual smile, took a sip of coffee, and then announced that she wanted to have a big party—not in a week but the following year—to celebrate our thirtieth in 2017.

My first reaction was a feeling of being overwhelmed. Planning a big party sounded like a ton of work. But just as quickly, I remembered what I asked Becky to do for me back in 2009, shortly after she was diagnosed.

Shortly after the prognosis, Becky and I were contemplating the future and how to go about dealing with it. During the conversation, I asked her to promise me that she would fight as hard as possible to make it to our thirtieth anniversary. I know that sounds selfish and, well, it was. Remember, I had planned on being married to this incredible person for at least sixty years. Thirty was nine years away and only the halfway point.

Looking back, I wish I had asked her to promise to make it to forty or fifty. I remember her smiling when I asked her to promise, and she simply replied that she would do her best. In that same breath, I also promised that I would do everything in my power to help her get there, no matter the cost, the time, or the sacrifice. She was my wife, my woman, my lover, the mother of my children, my best friend, my whole world. Giving every second of my life to help her fight and win as many battles as possible was my great honor and privilege, one I would do a million times more without hesitation if I could.

Becky grabbed her pen and we began brainstorming. We wanted the pastor who married us, the original church, the same reception venue, and as many other details as close to 1987 as we could get. The guest list would include family, close-to-home friends, and people on our Christmas card list.

As we began compiling the list, we soon realized we had to get a bit more selective. The venues we had in mind only had room for a certain number of people. And then there was the to-do list. It took us about an hour that morning to come up with a basic outline and divvy up the tasks.

I began sending messages and making contacts, while Becky came up with dress ideas, flower ideas, cupcake designs, and decorations. We both agreed we were going to keep it simple, but we both knew that there wasn't any way Becky was going to be able to hold her creative juices back. I don't know exactly how many mornings we sat in those chairs sipping our coffee and talking about that upcoming event, but I do know just how much I enjoyed them and how much I miss them now.

Today, these are some of the most precious memories I have from that period, just sitting and looking into Becky's beautiful eyes and listening to her sweet voice talk about things regarding "us," our marriage, our original wedding and all the wonderful things that were a part of our life then. It did my heart good to see her smile, to hear her reminisce about us, the things we used to do, the places we used to go, and all those magnificent times we were able to make love until the wee hours of the morning or in the middle of a sunny afternoon.

She would take those memories and use that energy and that love as fuel in her tank to help her keep pushing for that next April. I look back now and thank God every day that He dropped the idea of a party into her heart. Had He not, I know now that I would have lost her a lot sooner. The party became her focus and motivation to move forward. In hindsight, it was like an exclamation point to her incredible life of service, sacrifice, love and nurturing.

The farther and deeper we got into 2016, the more conflicted we became regarding Becky's prognosis. We knew the fatigue was getting to her. The frequency of down times was ever so steadily increasing, but there were still many good days.

Becky manned our office almost exclusively that spring, something she hadn't been able to do in a couple of years. She helped me plant an enormous flower garden, where she worked more and more as the seeds began to blossom. During that year, there were times that we actually thought this party would simply be a celebration along the way to many more.

23]   A LITTLE NORMALCY

One of the things that Becky and I liked doing together was regularly taking a day, usually in late spring, to shop for flowers, garden plants, hanging baskets and all the goodies that go with that. Our annual list of what to buy was bigger than ever this year, now that we had a huge, tilled space for planting.

The garden store we loved going to every spring—Marvin's Garden Spot—was a thirty-minute drive south, down by the town of Honor. After lots of time spent shopping, we would always take a side trip to the beach and stop for lunch. But most of the time was spent at the garden center with Becky doing what she loved more than just about anything else.

Our new garden was proving to be a wild success, with more vegetables than we could process, but Becky was determined to keep up. She made her usual huge batch of refrigerator pickles, bread-and-butter pickles, tomato juice and sauce, fresh salsa in varying degrees of hotness, and even some peaches she bought and canned. Together, we canned almost forty quarts of applesauce; not my favorite thing to do, but the work was an absolute blast because we were doing it together.

Becky's garden had a row of miniature gourds and a few varieties of sunflower plants that would end up over seven-feet tall. It was always a toss-up as to what was Becky's favorite flower, the daisy or the sunflower. Both usually ended up winning because each occupied a different portion of the season in their peak, and so she couldn't be happier than when she was reaching for the highest sunflower or sitting in a patch of daisies with her kids or grandkids, having their pictures taken.

As fall approached, Becky's physical strength was still declining a bit, but her tests and weekly blood work were giving us guarded optimism. In addition to planning our trip to Marvin's, she was already planning the decorations for one of her favorite holidays—Thanksgiving.

Oh, how she loved Thanksgiving. Becky was always irritated at the amount of press, retail focus, and family focus holidays like Halloween and Valentine's Day received, while Thanksgiving seemed to be nothing more than a day to eat like a pig and watch football. Becky was the most thankful person I've ever known. She had a heart of gold, a smile as big as the moon, and loved nothing more than making our home feel like you were walking into each season when you came through the door.

Because Becky loved being in the kitchen preparing amazing food and serving it with a smile to a family she loved and adored, we kept very busy doing the traditional holiday Thanksgiving and Christmas things and tried hard not to waste energy focusing on Becky's disease. There might be a need for an additional power nap here or there, or some increase in medication to offset the pain, or maybe just a quiet time in a chair while the daughters-in-law or my mom stepped in and took over for her so she could rest. But Becky vowed to keep at it.

Still, it broke my heart when she wasn't able to stand long enough, focus hard enough, or simply stay awake. It was moments like these when the awful reality of the long-term effects of the disease and the treatments became painfully apparent to all of us. It reminded us that Becky had already outlived her expiration date by six years. We hoped this was just another season that would pass, that she would beat the dour predictions, and we'd be off to another couple of years and new adventures.

By the end of Christmas, those hopes were dwindling. And then came unfortunate news, too, from another family member. A similar but more aggressive circumstance would remind us all of just what Becky was facing.

Sometime between Thanksgiving and Christmas, my aunt, Pat, went to her doctor to discuss an issue she was having with her breathing and some pain and discomfort in her chest. She was in her seventies, had smoked and drank a considerable amount in her former years, and was expecting the doctor to diagnose the discomfort as something heart related.

But after some tests and several visits, the doctor's report made our hearts sink. A melanoma she had removed on her arm six years earlier had come raging back and had settled into both lungs. She had maybe a month or two to live.

Aunt Pat handled the diagnosis with such grace and dignity; she even let my dad, her brother, know that she was going to beat him at something else—meeting Jesus before he did. She passed away in January just a few weeks after getting the news.

As we all sat around our place for Christmas, my dad, with a bit of a lump in his throat, said that 2017 could be a year when he would lose his sister, his mom, and possibly both of his brothers, since their health was also very precarious. We didn't think that Becky would be added to that list. Still, with the passing of Aunt Pat, we felt something shift, like a tsunami had started and there wasn't any way any of us could get to high enough ground to get out of its path.

After Christmas, the focus again shifted to the anniversary party. That and the daily routine of managing Becky's pain, hoping and—toward the end of January—praying for a good PET-scan result.

Planning the party continued to provide a good distraction. We spent hours of every day fine-tuning the plan, compiling music lists, creating decorations from scratch, designing a cupcake display, making 500 meatballs for the freezer, coming up with a full menu, and arranging help from friends who wanted to bear some of the load. All the while, my optimistic and courageous wife—despite feeling more and more fatigued by the day, dealing with more and more bone pain, nausea, and overall weakness—just kept plugging away as only she knew how.

24] ONE LAST ADVENTURE

Before I continue, I'd like to take one step back—to the summer of 2016. I was antsy and wanted in the worst way to take Becky on the trip of a lifetime. Becky just didn't have the wherewithal to plan anything away from home, so our bucket list sat unused. But the idea of a trip was something I just couldn't give up.

After a while, and simply because I think she was getting tired of hearing me talk about it, she agreed to let me go shopping for an RV.

Years prior, we had sold a fifth-wheel camper because Becky couldn't ride in the pickup for long periods without enduring excruciating bone pain from not being able to stretch. I knew that if we were going to pull off an epic journey, it would have to be in something where she could rest while I drove. A Class-A motorhome seemed our only option, and so I began scouring the Internet for deals.

I eventually found an RV for sale downstate, near Detroit, and we took a day to travel to get it. After arriving to meet the owner, a gentleman named Carlo, it became clear from the conversation that God had His hand in this whole process. Carlo took one look at Becky's bald head, then shared his own story. Just a few years earlier, after cancer had taken his wife, he told us how he had purchased the RV to spend a few years on the road recovering from that loss. By the end of our visit, we made an offer. Carlo threw in a very valuable recliner in the motorhome along with every possible repair part and tool, plus multiple tool boxes. Carlo even threw in a new propane grill.

During this time, daily fatigue had become more and more of an issue for Becky. We were still making our monthly trips to CTCA. So on one such trip, we took the motorhome to test it out before we left on a longer adventure.

The vehicle worked perfectly. Becky could stretch out anytime she needed in a queen-sized bed while I drove. We stayed in the RV instead of a hotel, parking in a lot next to the hospital. We had our own generator, shower, water, and cook stove. We also took the dogs, and lived just like we were at home. The purchase of the motorhome was proving to be a great decision. We got excited about a longer journey, and Becky gave me the go ahead to plan an autumn trip to the Grand Canyon in late October, just a few weeks away.

I looked at the extended forecast and it was perfect. We had another appointment at CTCA and got the okay from her oncologist to take the Grand Canyon trip. We stopped to visit with Andy and Jessica in Illinois, and a couple of days later we were on our way. I was in my element; I was finally able to have my queen next to me while I whisked her away into the sunset, literally, as we headed west.

It rained an entire day on the drive out, then sprinkled about an hour when we first arrived at the campground on the canyon's south rim. But the rest of the two weeks was sunny, with perfect temperatures and blue skies. Becky was a trooper, even though she was tiring more quickly each day. In the park, we explored every possible nook and cranny that her legs and energy would allow. Then, at night, we would retire to the motorhome where we watched our favorite movies while snuggling in bed.

It was a trip we wished would never end. We loved being out there together, exploring, just the two of us, with nothing to do except be together and take in the grandeur and expanse of one of the most incredible places on Earth.

After spending a week in the Grand Canyon, we made our way up to Arches National Park in Moab, Utah. This was another epic trip, and Becky actually felt good enough that day to take a nearly two-mile hike to see the famous Landscape Arch. At the end of the day, she was pooped but very proud.

Finally, heading home, we again stopped at Andy and Jessica's followed by another visit to CTCA. During these final months of 2016 and early 2017, Becky's cancer reports were actually looking pretty good. Becky's tumor markers were dropping and her cancer activity appeared to be diminishing. We were cautiously optimistic. Not long after we were home, though, an infected port and sepsis sent us to the local emergency room. And just like that, we were again touch and go and looking death square in the headlights.

For the remainder of that year, a "two-steps-forward-and-three-steps-back" routine repeated itself over and over again. Even as I write this, I'm on the verge of tears, trembling at the thought of all she endured—the pain, suffering, torment and emotional distress. We had no way of knowing at the time, but these would be our final days together—the last Thanksgiving, the last Christmas.

It was only a few months from her death now, yet Becky wasn't giving up the fight.

25]   NO WAY OUT

A s was the ritual for nine years, January marked the first PET scan of the year, and every time it came around we found ourselves wondering if this was the one with the bad news. We'd been doing that now for more than twenty-five scans. In fact, on more than one occasion I asked if we were increasing Becky's cancer risk by exposing her to all that radiation for so long.

The answer: It's a balancing act; to discontinue the scans would open the door to being blindsided with metastasis to the organs. In other words, damned if you do and damned if you don't.

Waiting for the results was the hardest part of the tests. On this particular trip, we were extra nervous because of the rough patch Becky had experienced just a couple months ago—the infection that happened in November.

Becky's weight was still an issue, because she continued to lose it, and her fatigue and pain were still up and down. But to our pleasant surprise, the scan showed a bit of improvement and stability in all the labs and organ functions.

So, 2017 was off and running, and the anniversary party was ahead. We headed home with the good news and began planning another party first—this one for the Super Bowl—and also worked on our usual spring marketing materials for our business. Even in the face of a good scan result and supposed stable organ functions, though, Becky continued to struggle with fatigue, pain, a poor white blood cell count from time to time, and bilirubin levels that would tick upward, ever so slowly at first.

Time between scans was three months, and so March would be the next scheduled trip to Illinois. Boy, did it come in a hurry. Very little snow fell in February and March, so our drive to CTCA was uneventful.

Since our last visit, Becky had continued to visit the local lab in Traverse City every week for blood work. Over the weeks since our last visit, I noticed a fairly consistent yellowing of the whites of Becky's eyes. Her facial skin color also looked a bit jaundice. It irritated her that I would walk up to her and look for color in the corners of her eyes. But something was clearly wrong, and the only number showing it was the bilirubin. All the other tests were within range and good. So, we just scratched our heads and hoped we'd get some answers on our next trip to Illinois.

Becky's lab work showed a slight elevation in her bilirubin. But her PET scan in March was the best one in months, with tumor markers improved. Tests showed every single tumor in her liver, chest, and bones had shrunk, many by at least half. Imagine our excitement and elation at this news. We could hardly believe it, and I couldn't wait to jump on my phone and text the family as well as post to the blog the good news.

So, after nine years in and four chemo drugs, it appeared we were finally knocking down the cancer. Becky was going to be our miracle girl after all. She would not only make our party in a month, but she would make it in style and use it to start another ten years of kicking cancer's butt.

Our happiness would be short, however. After we returned home, Becky grew very sick with the flu. Then I got it, too … sicker than I'd been in years. Imagine the fun we were having: Becky also dealing with the side effects of the chemo and me feeling like I'd been flattened by a tank.

We had to get Becky's lab work done again that following Tuesday. With her feeling so lousy, we weren't terribly confident about what the report would say. But it turned out the results weren't too bad; just a bit of an uptick in the bilirubin but still within normal range.

Two days later, on Thursday, after seeing Becky throw up more than usual and watching her eyes and skin continue to yellow, I called CTCA care management and asked what we should do. We were told to get to the local emergency room as quickly as possible.

Just like other times we'd gone to the local ER, I had no confidence that our local hospital would treat Becky's issues adequately. They were always quick to remind us that she was dying. There was also the ER system itself; only once were we ever processed in under six hours, and that was when we walked in the door with Becky's white blood cell count at 0.4 (basically nonexistent).

This time, though, she received first-class and incredibly fast attention. I guess if you're really, really sick—like almost-ready-to-actually-die sick—things hit a higher gear.

In hindsight, though, it seemed to make more sense not to stay in the ER but to get in the car and drive to Illinois and CTCA—only seven hours away. I knew when she got there, she would be in the hands of her care team and get exactly what she needed, rather than waiting to be processed, tested, have this and that ruled out before they would start any kind of treatment. Her CTCA care manager agreed.

And so, we headed off. I was still dealing with the flu myself; my fever had spiked at nearly 103 degrees the night before. I let the doctor know and was informed that, when we arrived, I would only be able to drop Becky off and wouldn't be allowed back in the hospital. The drive south passed without incident. But when we pulled into the ER around midnight, I felt this wave of nausea as the flu came rolling back. On the drive down it was almost as if God had parted the waters of sickness, just like the

Red Sea, only to let the waters rush back again when Becky was safely inside.

An hour after we arrived, I received a text from Becky saying that her temperature had risen to 103.8-degress and that her blood pressure was eighty something over forty something—incredibly low, even for her. But another hour passed and she wrote to tell me her temperature had fallen to just over 100. She was being moved to a private room, but she told me to stay in bed—she was in good hands and knew I was feeling terrible—and wait to come up in the morning. Once again, she said, I had come through as her "knight and shining armor."

It was a late Friday night when we arrived, and it would be four more days before we would know that everything I had done was pretty much for naught and no one, especially me, was going to be able to help her this time.

Becky's GI team wanted to do a new test on Saturday. The test involved going down her throat with a scope and checking for possible blockages in bile ducts leading to and from the liver. Unfortunately, the schedule wouldn't allow this procedure until the following Monday, so it ended up just being the MRI on Saturday to see if the test was even necessary. She was also retaining lots of fluid in her abdomen, essentially waste that was collecting in her lower extremities. An MRI didn't show anything as far as blockages, but they decided to go ahead with the GI test on Monday to see if there was something, anything, that they could do to help the liver function better.

Despite all of this, I was beginning to feel better as the weekend progressed. Becky, however, only continued to feel worse. Her fluid retention was making it almost impossible to get up and walk, not to mention being comfortable in bed. The doctors had to keep the IV fluids going because her liver was pushing everything she was getting out of the blood and into the extremities, causing dehydration in the organs, brain, and other parts of the body.

This was a no-win situation for Becky, who had put on fifty-pounds of fluid in just five days in the hospital. Imagine lying in bed for a few days and being fifty pounds heavier when you got up to leave. Her legs were so weak and the fatigue level was high.

Monday came and her doctor did the procedure to help alleviate blockages in the liver. It was a fairly noninvasive test for Becky, and she was quickly back in the room and recovering nicely. Later that afternoon, as we sat side by side in her room talking about this and that, the GI doc popped in and wanted to discuss the procedure. He even had pictures. He began to explain that he didn't find any obvious blockages, consistent with what the MRI had shown, but he did place a stent in one of the valves just to see if that would help reduce the bile that was damaging her already weak and frail body. We both took in the less-than-chipper news, not saying too much and not really having questions at this point. Not surprisingly, Becky was exhausted, as was I, so we just sat and listened.

When the doctor finished, he walked toward the door and we relaxed a bit, assuming the visit was over. Before he stepped through the opening, though, he turned around and waved me over his way without saying a word. He was motioning to the hallway and wanted to talk.

My world stopped for a second. My heart paused and my breathing slowed to almost nothing. I'm not the smartest guy in the world, but in that split second, I knew what this conversation would be.

It was a discussion I'd feared having for nine years. But it was the first time since May 2009—the month of her initial diagnosis—that any doctor had motioned to me to talk in private.

Suddenly, I was scared to take a step toward the door. But I did, and I could tell by the look on his face that he would share unwelcome words—the kind of words that cause him to hate his job. He said he thought we only had about a twenty-percent shot at seeing any improvement in the liver function. He added that, while operating, he saw more cirrhosis and damage to the liver than anticipated.

"I'm sorry," he said, "but there really isn't any more anyone can do at this point."

I asked him how long he thought she had, and he handled the question in typical CTCA fashion, saying there was no way to know for sure. Becky had lived and operated so far outside the box for so long that no one wanted to predict.

So, I asked a different way. I simply inquired if it was going to be sooner rather than later. With a sad face, he acknowledged, "sooner."

There it was. For the first time since the phone call nine years earlier announcing Stage 4 breast cancer, there was the news that the end was near—that there was no stopping this brutal and out-of-control train. Becky had all but beaten cancer. The tumor markers and scans had nearly proven that. She had fought back after a devastating femur break. She had been victorious in two bouts of influenza, countless transfusions of blood to keep her alive, sepsis on more than one occasion, thousands of miles of traveling back and forth, bone pain for years, hair loss twice, vomiting, choking, and extreme weight loss. Now, with the numbers looking great, we should have been celebrating a victory.

But her liver was shutting down, and there wasn't a thing anyone could do about it. The only possible cure was a liver transplant, and she wasn't a candidate for that.

So, there I was, standing in the hallway, knowing I had to walk back in, sit down next to my battle-scarred wife, and this time tell her she was going to die. And there wasn't anything I could do, nowhere I could take her, no other doctors or hospitals or tests or drugs or anything that was going to change what was happening.

I walked in and told her what the doctor had told me. We both sat and held each other, not crying, not laughing, not talking, and not trying to brainstorm or reason. We just held each other in the quiet and surreal realization that the fight had come full circle. It was time to prepare mentally, physically, emotionally, and spiritually for the next phase ... the transition to Heaven.

. . . .

Tuesday morning came, and Becky and I wondered when she would be discharged, if at all. We had to see her oncologist first to discuss what options, if any, we had.

Becky had grown very close to her care team—and they to her—over the past two years. Going over the lab work, Laura tried to sound positive, but I could tell by her body language that she would have rather been on any other planet in the galaxy, doing almost anything else, that day instead of having the conversation.

Then it happened, the suggestion of one last chemo drug they could try.

There wasn't any mention of the drugs or procedures to help the liver. The new drug would only fight the cancer, maybe. I spoke up and asked about the GI doctor's diagnosis of Becky's liver failing; Laura confirmed that there was nothing that could be done for that.

Becky jumped in and asked a very straight-forward question about the odds of the new drug working:

"What kind of percentage are we looking at?"

"Fifteen to twenty percent for most," was the reply.

"But no help to the liver?" Becky pressed.

Laura nodded. And it was at this point that everything changed for Becky and me.

For nine years, every time a doctor looked at Becky to ask or suggest a possible next step, my wife would always and without fail look at me and ask, "I don't know, what do you think honey?"

Together we would talk it out, pray about it sometimes, sleep on it and together decide on the next step and go from there.

But not on this day. Not at this moment.

Without glancing in my direction, and without any hesitation in her voice or wavering speech that would indicate she was unsure or in doubt, she said, flatly, "No. I'm done."

If she only had a few days or weeks left, Becky reasoned, there was no way she was going to spend them in pain, in a car or hospital hundreds of miles from home or in bed dealing with brutal side effects of some new chemo drug. She wanted to be at home, giving and taking in as much life as she could, for as long as she could.

A few minutes later—after a tearful hug from her doctor and an assurance that orders for hospice would be put in back home—Becky looked at me with small tears in her eyes and a troubled look on her face.

"Is that okay, honey?" she asked. "Am I doing the right thing?"

It was almost more than I could bear, and every part of me wanted to get every doctor in the hospital in her room and come up with a Plan B. But I knew that's not what Becky needed to hear.

I knew how hard she had fought, how exhausted and beat up she was, and how at peace she was with regard to the next part of her journey. I also knew how troubled and tormented she was at the idea of leaving us behind to grieve and be torn apart by her absence in our lives. I knew right then that she needed my support and my strength now more than ever. She needed to know I would be okay.

Every part of my being knew I wouldn't, but I steeled my face and my voice with assurance.

So, we began the goodbyes to and from her loving and committed medical team at CTCA. We packed up, and—for the final time—began the long, quiet ride home to Michigan from that great hospital.

I was taking my wife home to die, and I was devastated.

26] WAIT HIS TURN

I brought Becky home from CTCA on April 5, 2017, knowing we wouldn't ever be going back. We had just been given the worst news possible two days earlier, April 3, which also was our oldest son Tim's birthday. I was bringing her home to live out her final days. My job now was to help her say goodbye to as many people as possible while also doing my best to keep her comfortable and at peace.

Due to her failing liver and the massive fluid buildup in her system, Becky labored intensely just to get to the car. At home, she struggled with basic things like walking, standing up, and getting dressed—all things she could do on her own before we left a little over a week ago.

Our main focus when we arrived home was to do all we could to make it to our anniversary celebration on April 22, just seventeen days away. Looking back on it now, if we hadn't had that party planned, I may have never brought her home from the hospital. Her condition had deteriorated that much. She was just that sick. The first couple of days at home were consumed with us trying to adapt to a new routine, a new level of care, and a new level of urgency to complete some of the anniversary plans on Becky's list.

As was her habit for the years I knew her, Becky started picking off the various projects one by one, albeit slower and less focused, but smiling and forging ahead nonetheless. Our kids were home the first couple of weekends after our return. They along with their wives and girlfriends were a monumental help in decorating cupcakes, cutting out tags, making table decorations, and putting together party favors.

The Tuesday after we got home, April 11, was our actual anniversary date. I stopped all visits on that day, even telling hospice that their initial consultation would have to wait, because Becky and I were going to spend the day together—just the two of us.

Each morning, it became more and more difficult for Becky to get up and find the energy and will to get ready. The fatigue and the toxicity in her system caused by her failing liver was slowly but surely beginning to weigh her down and affect her quality of life in a very noticeable way. We hadn't planned to do a lot on our special day, because we just didn't know what to expect from one day to the next. But that morning, as I got Becky around and dressed and got her legs under her, we decided to go for a drive and ended up at our favorite place for lunch—Hang On Express in Suttons Bay.

Close family friends owned and operated the restaurant, so the place was very familiar. We knew deep down that this was going to be one of the last times we were able to go out on a date, so we headed up there hoping to make the time as special and meaningful as we could.

Before going inside, Becky took my hand and we walked across the street to the jeweler's, who happened to be a lifelong friend of Becky and her family. I had lost my wedding band years earlier, and the one that she had gotten as a replacement quite some time back never really fit that well. Our anniversary celebration was just eleven days away, and as we walked toward Will Case Daniels' place, it became very clear to me just how important it was to Becky that I have a proper ring on the proper finger for our party. This was the last gift I would ever receive from my bride, but possibly the most precious.

Lunch was filled with lots of emotion from the family that owned the restaurant. They knew when they saw Becky just how sick she was and what was coming soon. It was all they could do to wait on us and hold it together. Our families have been very close for years, and the pain of knowing what was coming and not being able to do or say anything to make it better is more than most people can bear.

Becky had to get up before the food was brought to the table and head for the restroom because of nausea. She came back looking a bit relieved, actually feeling better, although still not very hungry. One of the things we learned at the hospital was that, as Becky's body began shutting down, her appetite and her thirst would eventually taper off and become nonexistent. This was very natural; her body just didn't need the resources anymore. But we were also warned that this phase tends to be very difficult for caregivers and family, as not eating and drinking goes against every natural inclination. .

Everyone knows that if we don't eat or drink we die. That is exactly what was happening to Becky. We didn't know the timetable or exactly how the process would unfold. But we both knew it was just a matter of days, maybe weeks, and that every passing day would offer an ever more-noticeable decline in Becky's health, body function, brain function, and coherency. A lack of appetite was only one of the glaring signs.

Despite this, we had a pretty good day, even if we did have to end our trip early so Becky could get home and rest. Driving home, I did everything I could to keep a smile, but I knew in my heart that I was celebrating the last anniversary I would ever see with this amazing woman. The thought of that was paralyzing to the core, and my heart was crushed all day long.

Looking back on it now, I'm not sure how I was able to even function. God's grace is the only thing that comes to mind and makes any sense. He was giving me just enough to do what I had to do so I could take care of Becky, take care of our family, and do all I could to help her reach the anniversary party that she had thought of, planned, and was determined to make.

During the week of our party, hospice was on the scene to evaluate Becky and determine what resources would be needed and when. I knew the day of the party would be long and exhausting for her, so they brought a wheelchair for me just in case she wanted to sit at some point during the day and simply enjoy the ride. Before the nurse left that Wednesday, the 19th, I took her aside and asked for some brutal honesty.

"Tonya," I said, "do you think Becky has a real shot at making the party in three days?"

Becky's condition was really that bad. Her ability to stay awake, focus, and do even the slightest of tasks was becoming laborious and more questionable every day. Tonya replied that she really didn't know how Becky had survived to this point. The only reason she could think of was the party. In her opinion, Becky had made her mind up that she wasn't going to miss that day ... not a chance.

I only asked the question because, secretly, I felt like there was still time to cancel and let all of our guests know it wasn't going to happen.

The decision was made to push ahead, and Becky smiled and promised me she was going to make it until Saturday. If there is one thing I had learned not to question, it was Becky's determination to reach her goals. And I knew how important the party was to her. I also knew that if we were going to make it to Saturday, it would probably be by the skin of our teeth.

Everything was finished and ready to go on Friday, the night before. As we settled into bed that night—the last Friday night we would do so—I snuggled up to Becky, wrapped my arms around her, and held her tight. For the past couple of years, going back to early 2015, I was in the habit of reaching over each and every night, multiple times throughout the night, and softly laying my hand on her chest to make sure she was breathing. There had been so many nights when we had gone to bed with her in such dire shape that I wasn't able to rest unless I knew she was still with me.

As I held her this Friday night, the night before our party, I began to whisper in her ear. If you should happen to see Jesus at any time during the night, I told her, please ask Him to wait His turn. I wanted her to tell Him that He could come back in twenty-four hours if needed, but please give the next twenty-three to me.

To this, Becky just chuckled, gave me a kiss, and said "okay." What she didn't realize was that I was being incredibly serious. In my mind, I was having my own conversation with the Lord. In my heart, I knew He wasn't going to take her this night, certainly not after all she had been through—all the struggle, sacrifice, planning, and care that had gone into making the next day the greatest day of our marriage. He just couldn't. There was no way He would let her miss it.

In just a few short hours, a church full of people and a reception with even more folks would be a remarkable expression of God's love. Who gets to do such a thing? Who gets to plan an anniversary party for thirty years knowing that it also is going to be a goodbye party where almost 200 of your closest friends and family bring their own closure to the loss of a precious life?

I felt as if God had a plan, that He was allowing this to happen in front of us all. I felt as if all the love, joy, and testimony that would be shared would have a monumental impact on countless lives as the story was told and retold, for weeks and months to come. This amazing wife of mine was being interwoven into one of the greatest demonstrations of love, grace, and mercy ever witnessed by folks who love and follow God. It was something we had always talked about. As we tried on more than one occasion to find reason, to wrap our heads around the "why" with this disease, it always came back to this: The "why" had everything to do with showing and demonstrating to as many people as we could—for as long as we could—just how much God loves us and cares for us.

In our minds, there is only one way to Heaven—a path that starts with repentance, acceptance, and an acknowledgment of the need to turn our lives over to Jesus while we're still alive and breathing. That is the one and only way we will ever see Heaven and spend eternity with God. There is no other way, and Becky knew it. I knew it then, and by the end of our celebration and the memorial a couple of weeks later, tens of thousands would know it as well.

Becky's life, and now her steady and noticeable death, were turning people's hearts into soft and fertile ground where God would be able to plant His love, His word, and His plan for each and every person that would be a part of it. This was what had put a smile on Becky's face for so long. This was why she was able to accept and carry this burden, and this is why God allowed it, because He knew he had a woman in Becky who could face this with dignity, grace, and a never-ending smile.

27]   WE MADE IT

On Saturday, I woke to the sound of the dogs stirring as they did every morning. After checking on Becky and being thankful that she was still with me, I got up and headed for the door to let the dogs out.

As I went about my business—taking my morning pills, getting the coffee brewing, feeding the pooches, laying out Becky's clothes, and going over the list of last-minute things to take to the church/reception one last time—it became apparent that Becky was going to need all the help and encouragement I could muster to get her out of bed.

Weeks before, she had bought a cute jean jacket to wear with her beautiful dress. But as I began to help her get dressed, we both realized quickly that getting this jacket on was going to be all but impossible with her extra weight. Becky had been taking a diuretic to help with the fluid retention and had lost nearly twenty pounds of water, but the swelling was still just too much.

To my surprise, and probably because she was too tired and fatigued, Becky didn't seem to mind not being able to wear the jacket. So, I quickly jumped to Plan B—another jean jacket from years ago that was a bit big but comfortable and complemented her outfit well.

She was so gracious and appreciative. I, though, was heartbroken that she wasn't able to wear the jacket she had chosen. Thankfully, my mom had gone shopping a few days earlier and picked up a pair of shoes with daisies on them that were several sizes bigger than usual. Becky had already purchased a pair and painted them to match our granddaughter's shoes, but there was no way these were going to go on her feet today. Mom actually bought two pair of different sizes just to make sure Becky had something to wear that matched her theme. What a huge smile that brought to my sweetheart.

After getting dressed, she had just enough strength to stand and put on some makeup. But then back to the chair she went. Her color was extremely jaundiced at this point, and no amount of makeup was going to hide it. This made her a bit self-conscience, but I convinced her that she was as beautiful as ever and that between all the bright colors of her girls' dresses and the amazing blue sky, she was going to be radiant in every frame of every picture all day. Becky just smiled like she always did and gave me a hug.

It was at this moment that a very profound and painful realization flooded my thoughts. Holding Becky, I began crying uncontrollably. This surprised her a bit; I had been on an emotional lockdown until this point. As we held each other, she asked me what was wrong.

The short answer: I was crushed. In that moment, I realized I soon would not be able to hold my wife again. I told Becky that the thought of never being able to hold her, smell, and caress her goose-bump-covered skin, was more than I could handle. In that moment, the reality hit me, and I was totally devastated. I just really didn't want to let her go.

· · · ·

Many weeks ago, Becky was on the phone with a customer of ours who also happens to be a professional photographer. Carrie was a young wife and mother herself. She and Becky talked a number of times and, eventually, a kind of friendship began to form. So, when Carrie found out about our anniversary party back when the event was still in the planning stages, she very passionately offered to take the pictures for us on that special day. No charge.

Back then, Becky and I had no idea we would be looking at the end of our journey together. I remember first meeting Carrie face-to-face for coffee, and she turned out to be just as amazing in person as she was on the phone, a true gem of a human being.

This would become even more apparent over the months leading up to our anniversary and especially during the weeks following Becky's death. Carrie went from being a mere over-the-phone acquaintance to a genuine friend and, finally, a person I consider a guardian angel. She and her family have seared a place into my heart.

It was Carrie who read one of my posts on Facebook in the weeks after Becky passed and, concerned I was thinking about suicide, called me that next morning to talk. Over the course of an hour and after heavy tears from each of us, she poured her heart into me in a way that I believe saved my life.

Truth be known, I had sat with a pistol in my lap on more than one occasion, thinking about how much I missed Becky and knowing that with just a quick moment of resolve I could be with her. I had convinced myself that God wouldn't deny me Heaven in this situation. The only thing that stopped me from pulling the trigger was my family. I could never put them through such a thing, but it didn't stop me from thinking about it. And so, to have Carrie on the other end of a phone allowing herself to be used by God was one of the most incredible moments in my life.

. . . .

It was Carrie's idea to meet at the reception venue to get some photos while Becky was at her strongest. What a great plan that was, and we were so thankful Carrie took the lead. Her husband, Chad, joined her as he often does when she shoots. He had his own camera, and between the two of them they were able to capture some wonderful moments on film, preserving the treasure of this day for generations to enjoy. (The cover photograph of this book is one such moment.)

While Carrie shot pictures of Becky and the kids, I strolled toward the parking lot to stretch my legs and take a break. Sensory overload, you could say. What my eyes were about to see can only be explained by a God who loves us, knows exactly what each of us needs, and wants nothing more than to bless us every chance He gets.

Across the parking lot, and only partially visible around other parked cars, was the grille and hood of my all-time favorite car—an original 1983 15th Anniversary Edition Hurst Olds, complete with a T-top. My kids thought I'd seen a UFO or something as I shouted and hollered.

There wasn't anyone around the vehicle, so I ran into the hall to see if I could find the owner. I learned that the owner of the car was also the father of the young man who had been helping us set up. But I couldn't find either of them.

After running from room to room, I chanced to look out a window and saw both of them leaving, about to get into the car. I forgot how fast I could run, and I successfully chased them down before they got away.

The owner of the car, Tom, graciously drove the car over to where Carrie could take some pictures of Becky and me standing next to it.

Why the big fuss? For starters, I was sixteen when this car was unveiled. In 1983, the Hurst Olds was prominently featured in many car magazine articles. My bedroom wall was covered with pictures of it. I eventually owned one of my own, buying it on impulse twenty-four years prior, only to just as impulsively sell it little over a year later. The first worst decision I had made was buying it (the car was more than I could afford at that time), and the second and even worse decision was deciding to sell it rather than get a second job and figure out how to pay for it. Had I done the latter, I would own a car today worth double what I paid for it.

So, when I saw this car again after so many years and on this particular day, all I could think of was how much God loved us both and just how special He wanted this entire day to be.

Becky and I had invited about 160 people to the party. The guest list included our family and most of our Christmas card list. We were overwhelmed by the turnout and show of support. Most everyone in attendance knew exactly what they were getting into when they made the trip to the church and reception hall that Saturday. Most had received word via Facebook, family, and friends that this was going to be the last time they would see Becky alive and be able to talk with her. Most knew just how emotional this day would be, and they made the trip anyway. For that, I am forever grateful.

What was interesting was how many friends stayed as long as they could, visited, and helped wherever they could. Equally interesting was how many family members left early, and the handful of people who told us they would come yet failed to show up. That's left me somewhat bitter. And someday I'll put it behind me. But for now, it still stings knowing some family and friends had more important things to do than spend the last moments of Becky's life with her.

During the party, I did my very best to make sure as many people as possible spent a few one-on-one moments with her. These were last conversations. Most everyone who sat with her knew it. As Becky's dad, Bud, made his way through the receiving line after the ceremony—where Becky and I waited to greet everyone—he shared six of the most humbling and powerful words ever spoken to me. With tears inching their way down his cheeks and his voice trembling a bit, he leaned in and said, "You are a man among men." I'm quite certain, amid all the comments directed at Becky, that he had no idea how precious those words were for me.

So, what do you say in a situation like this, with Becky and I sitting there as friends and family pass by? There aren't any words that help with the pain of the loss. There aren't any words that miraculously make things all better. No amount of time will somehow make the pain of what's coming less cutting. So, what does one do?

Simple: You just sit, hug, smile, hold hands, and tell the one you're with how beautiful they are, and thank them for being a part of your life. You encourage them to get to know Jesus, so there will be a reunion in the future. You encourage them to live their life to the fullest; you encourage the faith of the one dying by reminding them of just how glorious the scriptures describe Heaven. You cry together for a time. You hug as long as possible, and then you make eye contact—look deep into the other's soul—and you get up and walk away.

You do all this knowing that the life on this Earth is just a vapor, a blink. The real life lies beyond the last breath. Life begins when this one ends. That's how you speak to someone who is dying.

. . . .

As sad as this day was on one level, it was a stunning opportunity for those who accepted it. After all, how many people get to bring closure to a relationship while still living? How many people have the opportunity to ask for forgiveness and to forgive others? How many people ever get to say goodbye in person to ones they love?

While it was happening, it seemed like the perfect thing to do. And I know in my heart it was, no doubt. But in the four months since losing Becky, I keep going back to those final two weeks and wishing that I would have had more one-on-one time with her. Wishing I had taken a few days uninterrupted for myself to be with her, just the two of us. Regretting not having those hours and those minutes like so many others did. What was I thinking? Why didn't I realize that she was going to use up her final hours and energies with everyone else?

Deep down I knew the answer. Those closest to Becky needed that time more than we did. Becky and I had 32 years of the very best life and marriage we could have imagined, and we both knew we'd be seeing each other again soon in Heaven. We didn't know that for sure about some of those final visitors, and so it became important to spend those final days with as many as possible ... to help show them the way to Jesus, to help touch their hearts at a very deep level, and to help imprint the map to Heaven in their minds long after Becky was gone.

I was also jealous for the time our sons were getting with Becky, one on one. But I didn't succumb to that. Instead, I did all I could to stay out of the way and let each of them bring closure with their mom the best way they could. This was their time, not mine. This was their final chapter with Becky, and it needed no part of me or anyone else in it.

As one after the other sat and held their mom, crying, saying goodbye, begging God for more time and trying so hard to wrap their heads around what was taking place, I found myself sneaking behind closed doors to wipe away tears. Stephen was outside on the back deck with Becky for quite some time. He told me later that he had let his mom know that he would be returning in a couple days to see her.

"Stephen," she said. "I love you."

He knew what she was really saying—that she knew she would be gone before he got back. That was more than he and I could bear. He had to leave to get back to work, but his heart was crushed, as were those of his brothers as they and their families each said their goodbyes and walked out the door to get on with their lives.

This is exactly what Becky wanted, what she needed, but it was unbelievably horrible at the same time. I was watching and listening to conversations that shouldn't have taken place for decades to come. I was witnessing young sons trying to tell their mother how sad they were that she wouldn't be there to be a grandma to their kids. How sad they were that each of them was going to miss growing old with her and getting to know her as an older grandma. I've never witnessed or been a part of something so deeply painful, and I hope I never have to again.

. . . .

Monday evening, the 24th, just two days before she died, I helped Becky post her last Facebook entry. You can only imagine how difficult it was in getting through this, knowing the finality of what we were doing and why. But Becky being Becky, she took this moment and made it about everyone else.

"My honey is putting this post on here for me today. This is something I wanted him to do when I couldn't any longer. If you're reading this now, it's because the toxins have finally gotten to the point where my silly brain just doesn't have enough to do what it needs to do. Kind of stupid but what can I do? This will be my final post on Facebook as I settle into my honeys arms and get ready to go meet Jesus, face to face. I know Him pretty good already but I can't wait to hug him. What an amazing friend He's been through all this and I'm so thankful to see glimpses of Him every time I look at each of my handsome boys, sorry, Men.

"There's no possible way I can even begin to thank every-one who impacted my life. All my friends at so many differ-ent points of my life. My family. The amazing customers I've been so blessed to talk with year after year since 2006. You all have made my life so great and hopefully, at least once

or twice, here or there, I've let you know how special and precious I always thought you were.

"If you know Jesus, I'll see you again.....In a blink right? If you don't know Jesus, please, please, please get to know Him. He loves you so much. He's waiting with open arms for you just like He is for me and I sooooo want to see you all again. I promise, you won't regret asking Him to become part of your life. I'm not talking about becoming part of this church or that church, this religion or that one. I'm talking about Jesus, just as He is, with no strings attached and nothing but love for us all. The other stuff will come, but Jesus is the most important part of it all. I love you all so much and so wish I could grow old with each of you and share grandma stories but it's not in the cards. I've got it pretty good though. From what I've read and what Jesus has put in my heart, heaven is a pretty spectacular place and I'm pretty sure I'll be taken good care of.

"Don't know how to end something like this so I'll just say this.....slow down, see the amazing gift you have in your spouse if you're married, love your family, treasure your children, adore your grandchildren and bake some cookies, watch some birds and listen for the joy. It's all around each of you. Bye bye."

28]   DON'T WALK, RUN!

A short time after Stephen went home, the Monday after the party, hospice arrived with the bed we had ordered to place in front of the living room window. Becky wanted to be able to look outside as long as she could, and I wanted to be able to see her every minute of every day no matter what I was working on. I didn't want her hidden in the bedroom all by herself, left to die alone. She was going to be with me and me with her for as long as we could make it last.

Becky was completely exhausted at this point. She wasn't eating or drinking, and the symptoms of the toxin levels rising in her brain were beginning to show. Monday evening, while on the phone with Andy, she actually forgot who she was talking to and had to ask me who was on the phone. I knew that Andy, in Illinois, was devastated and heartbroken at the reality of what was happening, knowing he couldn't do a thing to help. None of us could.

Earlier that afternoon, after the bed had been set up and Becky was resting, David got home from work. He walked in the door as he usually did, with a big smile and a hello, greeting his cats and our dogs. As he walked in the dining room, having a full view of the living room looking toward the front window, his eyes landed on his mom laying in the hospital bed and it was at this moment, after nine years of holding it together, after weeks and months of being the encourager and smiling his way through the pain and the reality of what was happening, that his world came crashing down.

David turned around and ran outside as quickly as he could get there. I found him sitting in a chair on our front porch, crying like he'd never cried before. There was something final and impending about seeing Becky in that bed, next to the window. We all knew we would be at this point eventually, but now it was really happening. Now it was undeniable. No amount of smiling, deflecting, or distractions were going to make it go away. Becky was lying in the bed, by the window, almost completely unconscious. She was preparing to die.

It took David an hour or more before he could walk into the house and enter the living room. He had to walk directly past the bed to get upstairs to his room. It was all he could do to make those steps, but he did it, and later that evening he would spend some time at Becky's bedside talking with her, holding her hand, and sobbing uncontrollably. Somehow, I had managed to again put my heart and my emotions on auto-pilot and do what had to be done. But I knew my moment was coming, and soon.

. . . .

Our son Tim, his wife Teia, and the girls came over for a visit. The girls climbed in bed with grandma where they sang songs and snuggled. After they left to go home, Karie and Tammy came out at my invitation to sit and visit Becky one last time.

Over the past several years, these two precious ladies had become two of Becky's very best friends. The three would meet regularly for coffee and sit together at basketball games (all of their sons were close friends). I know how much this visit meant to them and to Becky, and it was such a privilege to sit and listen to best friends have a conversation filled with love, great memories, and genuine gratitude for the lives they shared.

It was about 9:30 that night when the last folks had left, and it was just Becky and I and the pooches. She was exhausted, fatigued, mentally fuzzy, and ready to sleep. She had used up everything in her tank on friends and family, and there seemed to be nothing left for me. No more words. No more "I love yous." No more hugs, kisses, or anything. In just a few short minutes she would enter what would be her final sleep.

I didn't know this at the time. I was puttering around doing the chores: working on funeral details, gathering pictures, picking out clothes for the next morning, etc. With Becky's bed in the living room, I was able to do all of this and still listen to her breathing and watch her chest rise and fall. These things were the extent of her communication, and I didn't want to miss a moment.

After a while, I pulled the recliner next to her bed, got my pajamas, and curled up in the chair next to her. I laid my arm along hers, grabbed her hand, and laid my other hand directly over her liver.

As I'd mentioned, Becky and I, together, never once prayed for God to heal her. We always trusted Him to do what He was going to do, and put our faith in that. That night was different, however. Lying next to Becky, I was overcome with the desire to cry out to God one last time.

As I put my hand on her abdomen, I pleaded with Him that if His intentions were to heal her, please start soon and show me a sign so I could change my focus and help bring her back from the brink. If not that—if His plan was to take her home—I asked only that he please do it quickly.

"Please," I asked, "don't let her lay here and suffer for days and weeks."

I quieted myself after a bit, still holding Becky's hand, and waited. As each minute passed, I felt a peace come over my heart until I felt like I knew what the plan was. I knew I was holding my wife's hand for one of the last times in this life. I believed in my heart that God was going to honor my prayer. Why wouldn't

He? All I had to do was look at the past nine years—and especially the last three weeks—and know that He was going to finish
this story, finish this life in amazing style. I just knew it. I just
had no idea how amazing it was going to be.

. . . .

A few hours later, I was awakened by the most beautiful sun-
rise I had seen in months. My sweetheart was still with me. It
was Tuesday, just three days since I had danced with her at our
reception. Just three days since she had danced with each of her
sons and just three weeks since getting the news that there was
nothing left to do.

Where had the time gone? Time, now there's the real enemy.
You often hear of how fire or water or bacteria are the most
destructive forces on the planet. None of those holds a candle to
time. Time waits for no one. No matter how good or horrible a
moment, time chews those moments up. The strange part is how
we think the precious moments disappear in a vapor while the
painful moments seem to linger forever. No matter how much
time we have, it's never enough. And no matter how good of a
steward we are with that time, we are always left feeling that we
could have—should have—done better.

Becky was sleeping fairly peacefully, resting comfortably, her
breathing steady. I busied myself with a few morning chores,
then sat by her side and began talking. They say that the hearing
is the last thing to go, and so I believed she could hear my every
word. I was about to get a confirmation that she was listening.

At one point, I squeezed her, kissed her on the cheek, and
asked a simple question:

"You know I love you, right?"

And to my grateful surprise, Becky deliberately took a deeper
breath and groaned an affirming, "Ah hah."

These were the first words I had heard from her in more than
fifteen hours, and I cried, deeply. She *had* heard me. She was

listening, and she knew I loved her. I can't adequately describe how this made me feel. Becky was still with me, still connecting to me and my voice, even as she lay there staring into eternity.

. . . .

Our hospice nurse and an aide came by the house midafternoon to help change Becky's clothing, give her a sponge bath, address a bedsore, and make sure I had everything I needed. I was standing at the foot of the bed while she worked.

As the aide was in the process of adjusting the new clothing, Tonya looked at me and said, "It makes you sad, doesn't it?"

"No," I said. And I really meant it. "If she was eighty-years-old, I would be sad. She's only forty-eight. This makes me angry."

Tonya agreed, and we both shed some tears as we did our best to get through this step.

. . . .

After they had gone, later that afternoon, I got a phone call from Stephen. He was back home in Westland, near Detroit, and was calling to see how his mom was doing. I was holding Becky's hand and sitting next to her in my chair, and so I put him on speakerphone so I didn't have to hold the phone to my ear.

Stephen began to tell me about his time with Becky the day before. During their conversation, he said, she had told him how sorry she was that he and his brothers had to see her like this.

Becky looked as if she were sleeping. But she was listening, and I can only guess she thought Stephen was in the room with us. Suddenly, she sat up in bed and began crying out that she didn't want him to see her like this. She wanted him to go, to get out of there so he wouldn't have to be a part of it. She was so agitated and emotionally charged. Her sudden waking from what I thought was a sound sleep was so surprising, I abruptly hung up on Stephen and jumped to her side, grabbed her, and hugged and kissed her until she finally settled down.

It was at this point that I grabbed the hospice care package out of the refrigerator that had arrived a few days before. The kit contained morphine and another medication for agitation. Clearly, I reasoned, it was time for the agitation medicine, which didn't take long to kick in.

Becky was soon resting again with soft and steady breaths, and I went about my routine—working on the details for the visitation and the memorial service—while she slept. As the late afternoon approached, I climbed back in my chair next to her and held her hand once again.

I began to talk to her some more, gently took a sponge to her dry lips, and patted her warm forehead with a cool, damp towel. I don't remember the exact words I spoke to her during this time. I only wanted her to hear my voice and know she wasn't alone. I also wanted her to know it was just the two of us; obviously, this was something that was important to her. I didn't want anything hindering her from letting go and allowing herself a peaceful and glorious transition to paradise. But again, at one point, I asked if she knew I loved her. And she took another deep breath, uttered another "Ah hah."

Later, I found myself wanting some company. I took a chance and called my dad to see if he might come over to chat. I wasn't looking for answers. I just wanted to take a break and talk to someone about simple, everyday stuff. I knew talking to my father would help, and I also knew that—if I needed—I could ask him to leave at a moment's notice and he wouldn't think anything of it. He's always been a calming force like that, and this was one of those times that I just needed a quiet, calm, and empathetic face in the room.

After he had left, I decided to get ready for bed. Sliding the chair back over beside Becky, I sat and took her hand. I began talking, quietly, and that's when she began groaning. It was the same type of groan I had heard on numerous occasions over the past nine years. I knew it meant she was dealing with extreme pain, so I administered the agitation medicine and waited several minutes hoping it would help. It didn't. Becky's breathing came faster. Her heart rate and the groans became louder and more intense.

I called the hospice hotline, and got a quick return call from the nurse who instructed me to give a dose of morphine, wait fifteen minutes to see if it helped, and then call her back. Twenty minutes later, I called to report that—despite the dose—Becky's pain seemed to be getting worse. If these were to be her last minutes, this is not how I wanted it to go.

The nurse instructed me to give another dose of morphine, and told me she was on her way to the house. I was already feeling as if I had failed; Becky was in pain. I wanted to spend these last moments, just the two of us, and now the nurse was en route. David was upstairs, sleeping.

As I waited for the nurse, I did the only thing I could do—hug and rock Becky while telling her softly to just hang in there for a few more minutes. We were going to get the pain under control and make her feel better. I knew she heard me, although my words didn't seem to help mask her discomfort.

Twenty minutes later, the nurse arrived. Over the next hour, she was a calming force, very kind, compassionate, and professional. It took almost an hour to get Becky's pain under control.

This part of the ordeal began around 10:30 p.m. It wasn't until almost 3 a.m. Wednesday that Becky was finally comfortable and resting again. As she settled in with me holding her, whispering words of affirmation and comfort into her ear, Becky's breathing became increasingly short and shallow.

As I cradled her head in my arm, I knew the time was here.

"Sweetheart," I said. "Remember what I told you about asking Jesus to wait His turn last Friday night? Well, change of plans. If you're seeing Jesus right now, if you're seeing anything that resembles what Heaven might be or what Jesus might look like, don't walk, run! Run in that direction with everything you have. It's time for you to go be with Him. I'm going to be just fine, and I will be seeing you again soon enough. Run, run to Him now, Sweety."

Within ten seconds of me saying those words, and while the nurse was in the kitchen preparing the next dose of medicine, Becky took one final breath and let her head fall into the crook of my arm. She was gone.

In that moment, I had been awarded the greatest honor any loving husband could have—to lead my wife into the outstretched arms of Jesus. I literally felt her spirit release, let go from her mortal body. It's an experience I will take with me all the way to Heaven myself when it's my turn.

I'm reminded of this moment now on those days when I find myself getting angry, depressed, and even thinking stupid thoughts of just ending it all to go be with her. I had been blessed with precious years of time with Becky, extra time that allowed us to throw a going-away party where dozens of people came to say goodbye. And then—just when I thought I couldn't be more blessed—God allowed me to help guide my precious bride into the arms of her savior.

As I stood there holding her, the nurse came back to my side, put her hand on my back, and together we watched the heartbeat in her neck deliberately slow until it stopped. The nurse noted the time—3:15 a.m.

My sweetheart, my bride, and my lover was gone. I had seen and felt her heartbeat for the last time. Never again would I hear her voice, hold her warm hand, or dance with her to our favorite song. Never again would I make love to her, take a walk on the beach, watch a sunset, or calm her fears as she lay in a hospital bed. She was gone, and I was left with a shattered heart.

I had a very vivid picture in my mind of Becky standing next to Jesus, Him holding her hands and welcoming her into His presence with the words, "Well done, thy good and faithful servant."

It's this memory that sustains me today, one that keeps me sane and hopeful. Not bitter. For 11,778 days, I was Becky's husband, best friend, and lover. We were made for each other, but she was never mine to keep. And in that moment, she was gone—gone back to the one who created her for me in the first place.

Rest easy, my sweetheart, in the ever-loving arms of our king.

29]   THERE GOES MY EVERYTHING

A couple of minutes after Becky slipped away, I stood in the living room staring at her body as it rested in the bed. As I gazed upon the scene, an overwhelming and complete absence of fear enveloped me like a warm and comforting blanket. It was a feeling I'd never felt before or since.

When Becky died, I felt like my own life would stop. I expected to collapse onto the floor and be nothing more than an empty shell myself. To my disappointment, I was still alive and breathing. Only Becky was gone.

I also was painfully aware that, in that moment, my life as I had known it for thirty-two years was gone forever. It hadn't simply changed or shifted gears. It wasn't being reprioritized or adjusted. In a blink, the life I had known was over, and I had absolutely no idea what to think, how to feel, or where to turn. All I could do was stand and stare.

The nurse had about twenty minutes or so of paperwork to do, and I had some phone calls to make. The family at the funeral home had told me to give myself an hour before calling them, and so that's what I did. I used that hour to call parents and close friends and let them know what had happened.

Everyone knew this was coming. But it was still gut-wrenching to each person as I uttered the words "she's gone" to one, then another. As I was going through the motions, I kept thinking this had to be a dream, a nightmare of sorts. Surely, I would wake up in a cold sweat, reach over to lay my hand on her chest, and feel her alive and breathing just like every other time the past several years.

Even now there is pain, an intense and unrelenting sorrow in the core of my being that will not go away no matter how hard I try to suppress it. It must be like what sinking in quicksand feels like: in struggling to get out, you find yourself sinking faster; slow down, try to relax and focus on something else, and you're still sinking, still trapped, completely helpless, and unable to break free.

Nick and Ranve, the brother-and-sister owners of the funeral home, arrived at about 5 a.m. What a thankless job they have, but, oh, so important. The two performed their task with the utmost respect, tenderness, and genuine love for Becky, me and my sons. They handled Becky as if she was a princess and created an atmosphere of honor and dignity in a room that had been filled with pain and suffering.

At one point, Ranve gave me a hug, and I can't fully convey how much I needed it, how much I appreciated the calming presence of her and Nick and their tears. Nor can I ever thank them enough for helping to make the most agonizing of moments in a person's life somewhat bearable.

After carefully placing Becky's body, now in a closed body bag, on a portable, gurney-like bed, they gently rolled her out to a waiting vehicle. Goodbyes were exchanged, then Nick and Ranve got into the SUV and prepared to leave just as the sun peaked over the eastern skyline.

That's when my breakdown moment happened. I went inside, closed the front door, and stood staring out the glass as Nick put the car in drive and began to slowly accelerate down our long driveway toward the road. Watching the vehicle depart and knowing that the body of the woman I loved was inside, I was overwhelmed by grief, pain, sorrow, and loss. I fell against the doorway and wailed uncontrollably.

Three weeks ago the doctor told me that my sweetheart was dying and that there wasn't anything anyone could do. I just swallowed, took a breath, put my head down and began doing everything I could to get Becky through each day for as many days as possible. I hadn't allowed my mind to imagine this moment in detail yet. Oh, I had thought about life after Becky many times over the past nine years, but our hearts' defenses won't allow us to completely enter that place while our loved ones are still here. But now, as she disappeared into the morning, the full reality came crashing into my world and nothing was safe. Not my mind, my heart, my soul, my dreams, my imagination, nothing was off limits to the destructive power of this intense pain.

David walked up behind me and, without a word, placed his hand on my shoulder. He knew the weight of insurmountable sorrow I was feeling. In that moment, I had no desire to take another breath, no desire to ever feel happy or joyful again. It was my hope and prayer that my heart would stop as I leaned my head against the door and watched the tail lights turn out of the drive and disappear into the glory of the rising sun.

I walked back into the living room where Tim, David, and Jonny were now gathered, sitting, sobbing and trying to maintain a level of control. The four of us had no idea what to say, what to do, or what to think. Our other three sons, Andy, Stephen and James, felt even more helpless as they sat in their apartments hundreds of miles away and dealt with the loss with their girlfriends and wives. The cornerstone of each of these relationships and the matriarch of the family was gone. For nine years, each of us tried to imagine what this would be like and would we be able to handle it. For nine years, we lied to ourselves by convincing each other that we could. The lie was now exposed, Becky was gone and our worlds were wrecked.

30] NOTES, A JOURNAL, AND THE HEART OF GOD

Over the next nine days, I began to put together the final preparations for the visitation with the help of Nick, Ranve, family members, and good friends. As I've mentioned, I found myself going through every single notebook, journal, card, letter, and list of Becky's that I could find. Suddenly anything and everything that she had created—every written thought—seemed invaluable. I felt compelled to find and organize all of it, even the shopping lists.

This proved to be a very therapeutic thing—tough and incredibly painful, but therapeutic. Becky was an artist all her life. She could draw, write, paint, and create endless craft things without any effort. Even her writing was beautiful.

I started searching in our bedroom, where I eventually would spend an entire day. Not necessarily because there was so much to see, but because everything I found caused me to stop and weep. There were the notes she would leave on my pillow and the cards she gave me every year for different occasions that I saved in the drawer next to my bed. I read every one, each one causing a fresh wave of emotion. In some instances, it took me over an hour to regain my composure only to move on, find another piece, and have the process repeat.

Becky had been keeping a journal of sorts the past couple of years. The entries were sporadic and often no more than brief notes documenting how and when she was in pain, what medicines she had to take, or what hospital or doctor's office we had visited that particular day. Most if not all her journaling toward the end had to do with medical issues, and seeing this now made me heartbroken that her life was burdened with an unreal amount of pain and heartache.

I had initially decided on a quiet service with no plans for anyone to speak at the memorial. But as I read over her notes that first week, God began to deal with my heart. To honor Becky at the coming service, I realized there were five areas of her life that friends and family could speak about: her early years, prior to her and I meeting; her years as a young mom involved with Suttons Bay schools; her time when half of our sons were grown with two others still in high school at T.C. West; her role as a business owner/operator with me in our community; and finally, her role as my wife for thirty years.

In His way, God showed me the right people to ask and each one of them, without exception, expressed immense honor and eagerness for the chance. The only holdout was me; I was uncertain what I should do at the memorial.

It was a few days later when I found a notebook next to the bed. The book was filled with cute sayings Becky had either read or heard and then written down. But written there on the very last page was something else—a line of prayer she wrote, a line that would change my mind and make me realize I was the only one who could take all of the stories from family and friends and roll them into one focused and defined picture of her life.

Father, if this problem is needed to fulfill your purpose and glory in my life or another's, please don't take it from me.

I read it repeatedly as I sat there that day, crying. All at once, all these years of not feeling like we needed to pray for her healing or asking God for a miracle came into focus. Suddenly, it became very clear how Becky was able to conduct herself these past nine years in putting everyone else first while continuing to battle with a smile on her face and a seemingly endless supply of hope and encouragement for others.

This woman, my wife who had graced my life with her presence and love, suddenly became so much more. God had made her into a vessel to pour out His love and grace to every person she ever met. God had touched her heart in a way that very few ever experience. Not because God doesn't do that for them, but because few of us ever really yield to it and allow God to do it.

By writing these words in her journal, Becky had allowed herself to enter into the holy of holies while still alive on this Earth. She determined that God was going to have the last word and the last moment in her life and the lives of those around her.

After reading this line in her journal, I had never been more proud of Becky. All I could do was read it over and over and over. And eventually, as I found myself obsessed with this prayer, God broke through to my heart and let me know in no uncertain terms that I would indeed be speaking at her memorial and this prayer would be the exclamation point on an incredible life lived by a precious and selfless woman.

.   .   .   .

The visitation was magnificent. Nick and Ranve gave me the room to myself for about a half hour or so. Then the kids and parents joined me. Slowly, over the next three hours, the room filled, wall to wall.

I don't know exactly how many folks came but it was a fantastic turnout. What a joy it was to see so many people that Becky had touched over the years come out to pay their respects and share their love. I knew she was grinning in Heaven as Jesus stood next to her, pointing out all of the different ways she had touched each person. What a precious picture that is in my mind's eye, even now four months later.

Friends came from all over the country. And the flowers ... my goodness, the beautiful flowers. But just as Nick had promised, it was exhausting. Toward the end when the family was being encouraged to head out so the children and I could say our last goodbyes, Nick motioned me over to his office. He had his cell phone in his hand and wanted to share some numbers with me.

During the average funeral for a church in the Northern Michigan county where we live, he explained, around 700 to 1,500 people click the link on the funeral home's Facebook page to view the obituary of any given person. Once in a while, when the person is well known, the number of hits on the site might swell to 2,500.

Nick scrolled down the administrative page on the site, zoomed in on the latest number for Becky's obituary, and I almost fell over. Just fewer than 34,000 people had clicked on her obituary and read it. Not only that, but where most obituaries would see a dozen or two "shares" and a handful of comments, Becky's obituary was shared over 150 times, and there were at least that many comments on Nick's page alone.

How absolutely amazing and what a testament to her life and her impact on those around her. God's metaphor of the football stadium was indeed coming to pass. Ford Field has a capacity of 65,000. Becky's obituary—both the online version and the one featured in two local newspapers—had the potential to be seen by over a hundred thousand people. Nick used a metaphor of his own—that of a stone being thrown into a pond of calm waters and the ripples representing her influence and impact. In Becky's case, he said, it wasn't a stone but rather a very large boulder dropped from an incredible height sending waves, not ripples, for miles and miles.

I went home to an empty house that Friday night until the kids began to arrive. We had a few last-minute things to get ready for the memorial the next day and didn't have time to sit back and relax. Over the past nine days, I had only averaged about three hours of sleep a day, something that has continued to even now, four months later.

. . . .

The next day's memorial service was equally rewarding with some great friends putting on a huge feast. There was music, too. And it was perfect. The people who spoke all honored Becky and our family in such a touching and impactful way. The pastor's message of the cross—the only way to Heaven and ever seeing people like Becky again—was clear and on point. And then it was my turn.

I made my way to the lectern, my legs a bit shaky. My goal was to wrap the whole day into a beautiful picture of Becky. I guess I did okay. I brought folks to tears, caused outbursts of laughter, and in the end made everyone smile. I believe I made her proud.

My sons and I, along with a good friend, Barry, followed the casket out of the gymnasium and down the hallway to the back of the hearse that waited just outside the backdoor. Nick and Ranve placed Becky's body in the vehicle and then shared with us some mementos that we could take home: announcements, DVDs of the picture slideshow they had made, laminated copies of the obituary, the guest book, and the jewelry I had asked them to remove.

Then they got in the car and drove away.

The next couple of hours were spent visiting with friends and family. We shared stories, cried, and laughed, while inside I was doing my best to put a period on this chapter of my life. Soon, the party would be over, and I would be going home to an empty house and a life no longer with any purpose or direction.

Four months later, there are still moments when I find myself looking for the "why" in my day. I have lots to do, but often wonder what is the point of it all? Anyone who has lost someone dear to them can relate, I'm sure.

I don't know how many years it will be before I can piece this part of the puzzle together, but I'm learning to take life literally a minute at a time, hour-by-hour, and day-by-day. Perhaps one day, when I've grieved enough and the tears are few, I'll either be in Heaven with Becky and Jesus or I'll be writing the chapter in a new story with different actors and different adventures. Until then, it's simply enough to just breath and take one step and then another.

31]   BEGGING FOR A DREAM

Those first few weeks after Becky's death were brutal in so many ways. Thankfully, our minds have a built-in safety feature that only allows us to remember bits and pieces at a time and then only stores the non-catastrophic stuff in the front of our memory banks. The rest is sent deep into a place that is tougher to recall.

One of the things I found myself doing every night before I fell asleep was talking to Becky and to God, out loud, just as if they were sitting in bed with me. Each night I would beg God to allow Becky to visit me in my dreams and talk with me if possible. For those who haven't lost a significant loved one, this probably sounds silly. For those who have lost a spouse, especially after an extended marriage, you know exactly what I'm talking about.

Just a few nights after Becky left me, I remember crying myself to sleep. This would become a kind of daily ritual for weeks to come. Around 6:30 a.m., my two dogs woke me up to go outside. I remember waking up and being so angry and disappointed. There had been no dream, no communication, no nothing. Feeling empty and defeated, I called in the dogs, shuffled back to my lonely, dark room, and climbed back into bed.

I was jolted awake again at around 8 a.m., but this time by two very precious words spoken as loud as if someone was right there next to me.

"Hi, Honey."

That was what she called me—Honey. Every time she would answer the phone, or when I answered her call, the first thing she would always say was, "Hi, Honey."

I sat up like someone had electrocuted me, scaring the dogs in the process. The words were so loud and clear. I fully expected to see Becky standing there. Right then, I knew she had spoken to me. God had heard my prayer and allowed her into my heart to let me know she was okay. I sat there in bed, so thankful, feeling elated, overjoyed, and crushed, all at once.

It happened again about a week later. Only this time, I'd had a horrible evening and night before. I cried for a couple of hours and fell asleep completely defeated and in agonizing sorrow, begging God to let me go and be with her. About the same time in the morning after letting the dogs out, I climbed back in bed. Only this time I was crying again. I can't describe the pain, only to say that I just wanted it to go away. I just wanted to be with Becky.

I drifted off, falling deeply asleep, and suddenly, I heard her speak.

"I'm right here, Honey," she said.

My eyes jolted open and I jumped out of bed, certain I was going to see Becky standing there. She had to be there.

But, of course, she wasn't—not physically, anyway. Becky lived with God now, and God lived where our spirits reside, in our hearts. Not our physical beating heart, but the very core of our being. The heart we hear and imagine when we close our eyes at night with our heads on our pillows.

So twice now, Becky had come to me, and twice I had woken in amazement but was quickly shattered by the hard reality of her absence. Each time, though, was so incredible; I was excited to tell people about it. Each time added life to me and helped kick me over an emotional hump. The experiences also left me begging and dreaming for even more.

.   .   .   .

About a month passed, and I was losing all hope of hearing from Becky again. While cleaning out her dresser one day, I came across a silk negligée that she used to wear to bed on special occasions the first several years of our marriage. It was my favorite bedtime outfit—two pieces ... a top and some cute shorts. She had tucked it away in the back of one of her drawers.

I was so excited to find it, in perfect condition and soft and silky as ever. About that same time, I also found an old bottle of perfume she would wear once in a while when she wanted to light up my world. Instantly, I had a brilliant idea.

More than a few people I had talked to—widows and widowers who faced the same feelings of disconnectedness and loss after the death of their spouse—told me that they would take articles of their spouse's clothing with them as a way to remember how they smelled. I knew I would have a hard time with that; Becky didn't wear perfume very often.

But when I finally found that perfume bottle, I sprayed a bit on the top and bottom piece of her outfit and wrapped it around my neck like a scarf. I went to sleep like this, silly as it may sound, and four months later I'm still doing the same thing.

Once I began doing this, I found it easier to fall asleep. I still grieved the worst at bedtime. But the feeling was not quite as sharp. I no longer begged God to see her.

So ... it came as a surprise when Becky then came to me twice in a dream.

The first happened in early morning. Becky and I were sitting on a couch in a bright waiting room; she was cross-legged in the corner wearing a very cute and sexy lingerie outfit. We just sat and talked for what seemed like hours. I had my camera and asked her if I could take some pictures, and she happily agreed. Occasionally, we'd kiss and cuddle, but then we just went back to talking.

After quite a while of this, she suddenly got up, excused herself, and almost immediately I was transported to a table in a cafeteria somewhere. As I sat there, I noticed a waiter heading my way. He walked up to the table and handed me a pint of Haggen-Dazs Vanilla Swiss Almond ice cream—a treat Becky often brought home the first couple of years we were married.

The waiter handed me the ice cream and pointed across the room.

"Compliments of the pretty girl standing over there," he said. I looked and, of course, it was Becky. She smiled and waved before disappearing out the door.

I woke up and then sobbed uncontrollably. I couldn't thank God enough for allowing her to come and visit me. But I also couldn't get the image of her saying goodbye and walking away out of my mind.

. . . .

Two weeks later, Becky visited again in a dream. In this one, I was walking along the bottom of a massive row of stairs in what looked like a giant train station. The train arrived at the top of the stairs, and from there I heard someone calling, "Honey!" I looked up, and there was my Becky—young, vibrant, and beautiful as ever—waving for me to join her.

I ran up the stairs. But as I did, she disappeared through a door at the top. Dashing through the door, I heard her laugh with joy, then saw her run my way before jumping into my arms. We hugged and I held her up, kissing the longest and deepest kiss I could remember.

I slowly let her down to her feet, but had I known what was coming next, I would have never let her go. As her feet touched the platform, Becky gently let go of my hands, raised her head to kiss me again, then walked down toward the tracks. As she did, a train came grinding in, slowing but not stopping, as it approached where she was standing. In one smooth and methodical motion, Becky stepped up on the moving train, looked back at me waving, and told me goodbye.

Even now as I write this, almost two months since it happened, I can't control the tears. I had a feeling when I woke up that this would be the last time I would see Becky in a dream. This time, she was leaving for Heaven for good. I just knew it. She had come back one more time to make sure I knew how much she loved me and to let me know she had to go.

I lay in bed for hours that morning feeling paralyzed, devastated, relieved, yet happy.

It took me several days before I could climb out of the funk the dream put me in. The notion that I would never see Becky again until I, too, was in Heaven was crushing. I would have given anything to hear or see her again, but I knew that it wasn't up to me.

I also know now that she's just fine—young, vibrant and eternally alive—in the presence of Jesus. I just wish I could say the same for myself. Months have gone by, and here on Earth I still find myself feeling incredibly alone, walking through my days in a fog of intermittent loneliness and grief. Then at night, holding Becky's pajamas and breathing in her perfume, I continue to hope that maybe, just maybe, she'll come again to me in a dream.

32]   ETERNALLY YOURS, MY SWEET LOVE

This book has taken me thirty-two years and four months to write. The thirty-two years were the story-building years, and the last four months were simply the task of putting it all in words.

I never pictured myself a writer, per say. I've always had the gift of gab, but it wasn't until nine years ago—when I took up the task of writing a blog about Becky's journey with cancer—that I became aware of writing's therapeutic value. Writing those journal entries not only helped me but I believe also helped the online readers who were following our struggle.

I've lost count of the number of folks who have encouraged me over this past decade to write a book about our love story, our journey with cancer, and my life since. I was hesitant at first. Then I began to brainstorm chapters, and it was like God opened up a valve in my memory, allowing my heart to go back and piece together a storyline that afforded me the most amazing marriage to an incredible woman and mother who poured her entire life into making her sons' lives the absolute best and eternally rewarding they could be.

The past few months have been brutal. The grief comes in waves. For weeks, I've been propping myself up, pretending to be okay. I have devised distraction after distraction, thinking that—if I could only keep my mind occupied—I could put Becky away and move on like some magical movie moment.

A few days ago, I realized that there was no way that could happen, not now and maybe not ever. And since I've dropped my guard and allowed myself to just be in the moment, the moments have become painful and paralyzing. I literally can't do, think, look at, or remember anything without thinking of her and feeling the crushing loss of her presence all over again, multiple times a day.

What plagues a mind and a heart after losing someone like Becky are the regrets—all of the time I wish I would have spent together instead of working, driving all over the country, and being gone for weeks at a time.

Instead of bowling on leagues with co-workers or mountain biking with buddies or weekend-camping with friends; instead of the hours wasted watching news and being fixated on elections, or politics or other garbage like that; instead of the time spent worrying about finances; instead of those nights when she went to bed much earlier than me, by herself, while I stayed up watching TV, working on photography, or catching up on office work.

On all of those nights, I could have been lying in bed with her, just holding her and listening to her breath. That's the one that gets me the worst right now. What I wouldn't give to have her here just one more night.

I miss all the special meals Becky made just for me, because she knew how much I loved them. I miss the warm, fresh-from-the-dryer clothes she would lay on the bed for me on cold winter mornings. I miss the way she laughed at all my silly jokes and one-liners. I miss her soft and gentle touch, her smiling face, and her goofy interactions with our sons. I miss the walks on the beach, holding her hand and brushing her hair on evenings before bed, evenings that now seem sadly too few. I miss, well, everything. I miss everything about her.

Becky always made me feel better as a man and husband. The way she would always honor and respect me—never missing an opportunity to give me praise in front of our family and all who knew us. She always made me feel like the greatest man who ever lived and that she was the most blessed woman because I was hers.

But hands down, without a doubt, the most heartbreaking thing was Becky's radiant, captivating, and genuine smile. I've looked over thousands of pictures these past four months and am hard pressed to find one of her that doesn't show her smiling. As I write this, I've had to stop countless times and wipe the tears, especially, when I write about her smile and the void that now exists in my life without it.

Even during those painful and debilitating days leading up to her final hours, Becky's smile was always there. She was, without a doubt, the most optimistic, happy, cheerful, beautiful, and genuinely peaceful person I have ever known—an angel on Earth. When I look for meaning, a reason to explain why God took her from me at such a young age, it always comes down to this.

Becky was just so precious and radiant that He wanted her all to Himself, to smile in His presence, and spend her days loving on Him, face to face. I don't suppose I can blame Him. I just wish it didn't hurt so much.

I keep looking out the front window, expecting her to walk up the drive. I picture her sitting with me on the front porch and telling me all about her adventures these past several months. And the tears begin to flow.

Then one day, just a few weeks ago, as I looked down the drive, it occurred to me that she was doing the same thing in Heaven. She was standing at the window and gazing in our direction, wondering when we were coming to join *her*.

I've always known that this life is just a moment in time, a blip. We're just passing through. Now I see that there's no point in looking for Becky to arrive. Heaven is our real home. And, right now, I'm the one who is out of place.

AFTERWORD: THE THINGS I'VE LEARNED

The journey Becky took taught me valuable lessons about living as well as dying. I share this list in hopes that our experiences will prove helpful to the reader.

- Cancer doesn't discriminate. Sometimes you just get it, no matter how many things you do right.

- You make the best decision you can with the information you have available. Don't beat yourself up later about the path you took.

- Don't over-analyze something you know very little about. Make your decisions and live with the consequences.

- At the end of the day, after you've exhausted the resources available, look to Heaven and trust that God will see you through, no matter the outcome.

- Love your spouse as if today was his or her last day on Earth. One day it will be, and on that day, you'll be at peace.

- Learn to love with your heart and your spirit. That way, when the body fails and the soul is tired, the bond will not diminish, but become more clear and unbreakable.

- Terminal cancer is evil. But it can teach its patients and their caregivers strength, perseverance, and a deep awareness of life's beauty.

- I can find new love and someone to take my heart and bring healing and restoration. But my kids will never have another mom.

- How we live when we're preparing to die shows the world everything within our hearts. Becky's heart was pure gold.

- Once we realize that perfect healing is when we're in Heaven, in the arms of Jesus, we'll spend less time begging God to heal us now and just get busy living.

- The great thing that happens when we lose someone who holds our hearts is that all fear vanishes and life gets really simple.

- Start living off your bucket list now. Tomorrow is a pipe dream promised to no one.

- Grieving is nothing to be taken lightly, nor is it anything to fear. It is only to be experienced, one minute at a time.

ABOUT THE AUTHOR

Paul Wheelock is a fifty-one-year-old business owner and father of six sons. He has worked in the heating, ventilation and air-conditioning supply business and has driven trucks more than a million miles across the country. He and Becky started a pest control business in 2006 and it continues to grow and flourish. He enjoys photography, traveling the country to visit his children and grandchildren, and writing. He currently calls Leelanau County, in the northwest corner of Michigan's lower peninsula, his home and has lived in the area his entire life. His greatest hope is that people will find some joy, some comfort, and some hope in this story … and use it to fight their own battles.

ACKNOWLEDGEMENTS

This book would not have been possible without the encouragement and gentle pushing of a few wonderful friends and family. First, I would like to thank all of the many folks who followed my Caring Bridge blog, which tracked the nine years of our battle. That is where the encouragement to write this book began.

I can't begin to name everyone. But one couple I must acknowledge first is Scott and Tommye Solem. Shortly after Becky's passing, they helped me see the possibility of this work during a dinner at their house on Stony Point near Suttons Bay, Michigan.

My dad Don and his wife Jean as well as my mom JoAnne have each taken turns listening to me ramble on about the story and its progress, all with smiles and encouragement.

I also want to thank my cousin Sherry and her husband John for being the first ones to read my manuscript and offer up their heartfelt and honest critiques.

My first lunch meeting with Doug Weaver of Mission Point Press, my book publisher, was when I first really believed I had something of value. I would like to express my immense gratitude to him, Bob Butz, and Heather Lee Shaw, for their editing and design efforts. They found the priceless, true story within my manuscript.

My six sons have also been tremendous voices of encouragement regarding this book. Who they are—and the joy they bring to my life—come directly from their mom. I'm especially grateful for my oldest son, Tim. His work ethic, his drive, and his willingness to take over our business in the spring of 2017 allowed me the time and privacy to take on this project.

And now to thank the one who is responsible for each and every word on each page. Becky, my late wife, was the most amazing woman, wife, and mother. It's her love for me, our sons, our neighbors, and God Himself that made this book possible. I owe each memory shared on these pages, both joyous and devastating, to her beautiful life.

Thank you, Becky.

CPSIA information can be obtained
at www.ICGtesting.com
Printed in the USA
LVHW031629090223
739121LV00019B/841/J

9 781943 995608